T0275563

MODERN AND TRADITIONAL MEDICINE:
Conflicts and Reconciliation

Book Reviewers and Editorial Advisers

Prof. Umaru Shehu — Emeritus Professor of Community Medicine, University of Maiduguri Nigeria.

Dr. Y. Lawan Gana — Director Medical Services, Ministry of Health, Borno State.

Navy Captain L.M. Adams — The Officer-in-Charge, MRS DHQ, Mogadishu Cantonment, Abuja.

Navy Captain Y.D. Gunat* — The Captain Medical Centre NMC Onne - Port Harcourt.

Capt. D.O. Nabaida — The Commandant, NNSS Port Harcourt.

Pharm. Musa Umar — Chief Regulatory Officer NAFDAC North Eastern Zone Area Laboratory Complex Maiduguri.

Alhaji Musa Garba — President, Nigerian Union of Medical Herbal Practitioners, Barno State.

Pharm. Nuru Abdullahi* — Member, Pharmaceutical Society of Nigeria.

Mr Hamisu Habila — Senior Community Health Extension Worker (SCHEW) University of Maiduguri Teaching Hospital

---

* Now late (may their souls rest in peace).

MODERN AND TRADITIONAL MEDICINE:
Conflicts and Reconciliation

Umar Faruk Adamu

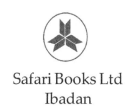

Safari Books Ltd
Ibadan

Published by
Safari Books Ltd
Ile Ori Detu
1 Shell Close
Onireke, Ibadan
Email: safarinigeria@gmail.com

© Umar Faruk Adamu

Publisher: Chief Joop Berkhout, *OON*

Published 2006
New edition 2013

ISBN: 978-978-8431-13-8

Dedication

To

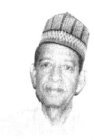

Professor Umaru Shehu, *CFR, FAS, FWACP, DFMC.*
A great teacher, medical scholar, professional father,
mentor, great Nigerian, and lovable man.

Formerly
* Professor and Head of Department of Community Medicine, ABU, Zaria.
* Deputy and Pro Vice-Chancellor, Ahmadu Bello University, Zaria.
* Director, Institute of Health (Otherwise, Chief Medical Director, Ahmadu Bello University Teaching Hospital (ABUTH).
* Provost, College of Medical Sciences, University of Maiduguri.
* Vice-Chancellor, University of Nigeria, Nsukka.
* Chairman, Board of Management, University College Hospital, Ibadan.
* Pro-Chancellor and Chairman, Governing Council, Bayero University, Kano.
* Chairman, Committee of Pro-Chancellors and Vice-Chancellors of Nigerian Universities (States and Federal).
* Visiting Professor, School of Medicine, North Carolina, USA.
* National Co-ordinator (Nigeria) and Director, Sub-Regional Health Development Office III, World Health Organisation (WHO).

Currently
   Emeritus Professor of Community Medicine, University of Maiduguri and Consultant Public Health Physician, University of Maiduguri Teaching Hospital.

Citation

The attitude of many an orthodox medical practitioner that he has everything to teach others concerning disease, health and cure and nothing to learn from them, is not just. Such an attitude cannot be reconciled with wisdom, intellect, scholarship and the spirit of scientific inquiry!

Similarly, the attitude of many a traditional healer of viewing modem advances in medicine with contempt and disdain, his refusal to follow the trend of changes sweeping across the world and his preference to remain primitive amidst modernity, must be condemned. Such an attitude will definitely isolate him and modern development will certainly bypass him and our bridge may not avail him!

Food for Thought

(Great Words from Great Minds)

"It seems paradoxical at a time when modern scientific medicine appears to be making giant strides, and enjoying unparallel prestige, that so much interest should be taken in traditional medicine in both developed and developing countries."

– Dr. Bannerman, Director WHO

"The medical herbalist is at fault for clinging to outworn historical authority and for not assessing his drugs in terms of today's knowledge, and the orthodox physician is at fault for a cynical scepticism with regard to any healing discipline other than his own."

– Penn R. G. (*Adverse Drug Reaction Bulletin:* No 102, 1983)

"We in the World Health Organization pledge ourselves to an ambitious target, to provide health for all by the year 2000. This ambitious goal is, quite simply beyond the scope of the present health care system and personnel trained in modern medicine. This is why the WHO proposed that the great numbers of traditional healers practising today in virtually every country of the world should not be overlooked. Let us not be in doubt, modern medicine still has a great deal to learn from these collectors of herbs."

– Dr. Halfdan Mahler, Former Director-General, WHO

Contents

Foreword I

The Nigerian population can be roughly divided into three major groups when it comes to patronage of health institutions. These are those who patronise only modern medical health institutions, (for example, hospitals, medical centres and pharmacy shops), only traditional health institutions, (like herbalist, bone setters, barber surgeons, religious healers) and those who combine the two.

The various controversies surrounding the supremacy of one practice over the other has been a subject of continuous discussion in this country over the last two decades. *MODERN AND TRADITIONAL MEDICINE: Conflicts* or *Reconciliation* focuses on the historical perspective of the two types of the medical practice, the various criticism of both practices and their limitations. The author painstakingly gave good suggestions on how to improve our traditional medical practice especially the herbal preparations with National Agency for Food and Drug Administration and Control playing a major role. He also reiterated the much-advocated need for the integration of some aspects of traditional health medicine into the orthodox medical practice. This he believes would cut cost and produce an affordable and sustainable health care to all Nigerians.

I strongly recommend this book to all Nigerians especially those who believe that the wealth of a nation and the administrative competence of its leaders should be determined by the health care of the populace and not the well-being of a privileged few. Additionally, I congratulate Surgeon Lieutenant Umar Faruk Adamu for a job well done and his contribution to the intellectual discourse of the country.

Navy Commodore Bola Sanni (Rtd),
Former, Director of Medical Services,
Nigerian Navy.

Foreword II

As a physician who is interested in medical history, I could not but welcome and appreciate such an initiative taken by Dr Umar Faruk Adamu in writing this book, *MODERN AND TRADITIONAL MEDICINE: Conflicts or Reconciliation*. The amazing aspect of this is that here is a young physician, with few years post-qualification experience and currently in active military service and yet still, he had found the time and the energy to write such a fascinating book. It is quite interesting to note that he has earlier authored and published other books on varying medical topics.

Having gone through the contents of this book, I knew that Dr Adamu had not taken lightly the task of writing this book. Considering his young experience in medical practice, one must commend his exceptional courage and foresight in research and scholarship. It is self-evident from his grasp and thorough handling of the issues raised herein that he had searched far and wide to avail himself of relevant current literature on the subject. There is, of course, a lot of literature to read on traditional medicine and modern medicine which describe the evolution of the two systems. This process has not been without problems over the ages and they are still with us.

In this book, Dr Adamu discusses the merits of the two systems as well as their limitations and shortcomings. Medical practitioners like ourselves who have been long in the health system, have experienced most of the situations which he has described. Some of us have engaged in the process of, if not reconciling the differences, at least in trying to establish an understanding between the two systems for the benefit of society. Progress in these directions has not been significant for the reasons which the author clearly highlights in this book.

The author has boldly made some rational suggestions

on how to overcome the suspicions and misconceptions which have developed over the ages between the practitioners of traditional and orthodox medicine. There is an urgent need to make a deliberate effort to inform and educate everyone including the community on the· two systems while the infrastructure for monitoring and controlling traditional practices in the country is being put in place.

Finally, while commending the efforts of the author on this book, I would commend that everyone, particularly those providing traditional and orthodox health services, should read the book. Dr Adamu deserves the support of all who desire to see the provision of affordable, accessible, appropriate and cost-effective medical and health services to our people.

Professor Emeritus Umaru Shehu
University of Maiduguri, Nigeria

Preface

Since the dawn of history, man has been puzzled by the sudden ravages made by diseases and has attempted in many ways to seek for cures for his ailments. Such cures have passed through various vicissitudes; from the earliest stages of superstition and witchcraft to the use of remedies sourced from religions, and gradually to the modern era of scientific enquiry and rational use of drugs. In spite of the spectacular advances made in the fields of modern medicine and the physical cure of disease, the war between man and disease is far from over.

The success of man in solving a problem appears to mark the beginning of a new one. For example, the control of infectious diseases in the developed world led to an increase in life expectancy. Man's desire for new pleasures became manifested through consumption of saturated fats, cigarette smoking, alcoholism, sedentary lifestyle, etc. These resulted in epidemics of non-communicable diseases such as hypertension, diabetes mellitus, obesity, bronchial asthma, cardiac diseases, peptic ulcer, stroke, cancers, renal and gall stones, etc. Age-related disease also became more manifest.

Furthermore, following the discovery of anti-microbial agents like penicillin and development of vaccines, diseases like small pox, louse-borne fever, and yaws were laid to rest. Many other communicable diseases were put under control. But while man on the one hand is saying *kudos* to scientists and trying to conquer his environment and disease, and assume dominion over the rest of creation as 'master of the universe,' the micro-organisms on the other hand, are unrelentingly reasserting themselves by developing resistance to anti-microbial agents. The excessive use of antibiotics and their irrational use has enabled several species of bacteria to proliferate dangerously and acquire resistance by undergoing.

some structural, molecular or chemical changes. Then new diseases and infectious agents emerged! Among which are the Human Immunodeficiency Virus (HIV) which sadly, provided ground for resurgence of so many diseases by reduced host resistance. The victory over tuberculosis, leprosy, pneumonia, typhoid, malaria and other infectious diseases now seems to be under threat. Without any cure in sight, the progress made by man in medicine could be at risk.

As the reality of these problems takes their toll on society, man continues, albeit desperately, his adventurous search for protection against disease and suffering. As a result, the use of plural medical systems is now a reality rather than a matter of theoretical debates and arguments. In Nigeria, the progressive devaluation of our currency coupled with an inevitable escalation in the cost of imported and locally produced drugs and medical facilities make modern health care services to the common man seem astronomical. Consequently, about 80% of Nigerian homes at one time or the other consult and patronise traditional medical practitioners, who provide cheap, simple but crude and sometimes harmful services.

In spite of this development, there is no official framework on the role of traditional medical practitioners in modern health care delivery. The existing policy of government is one of tolerance rather than integration of traditional medicine into the mainstream health care delivery in the country. The exception is the herbal medicine, which is recognised and even encouraged, but not effectively regulated by the government. There is now growing awareness of the need to regulate the relationship between the two systems of medicine prevalent in the country, in order to evolve and develop a comprehensive health system through which effective health care can be made both accessible and acceptable to the people. This endeavour calls for a multi-sectoral approach and close cooperation between agents of health care delivery, and between the many social, economic and political actors with the health sector playing the major role. This quest for mutual understanding and harmonisation of health care delivery has become more crucial now, more than ever before.

Surely, most of the developing countries are in need of inexpensive, and effective treatments for diseases. World Health Organisation (WHO) estimates that one-third of the global population still lacks regular access to essential drugs, and that in the poorest parts of Africa and Asia, this figure rises to over 50%. In these regions, some form of traditional medicine is often a more widely available and affordable source of health care.

In Nigeria, in view of the socioeconomic status of the country, the magnitude of the health problem and the limited resources, it is considered timely that any merits of traditional medicine ought to and should be viewed, reviewed or revisited. The challenge is to recognise and ensure that the health skills and knowledge of traditional medical providers are optimised. Thus, the concerted efforts of all are bound to generate intellectual profundity that will eventually determine the future of health care delivery system in the country.

Surgeon Lieutenant Umar Faruk Adamu
Directorate of Medical Services
Nigerian Navy.

Acknowledgements

If I have seen further, it is by climbing upon the
shoulders of giants – Sir Isaac Newton, 1600.

Just like the previous publication, I have literally climbed the shoulders of many giants to see the successful re-publication of this work. Although by no means a revised edition, efforts were made to modify the packaging and the cover design in order to give it a new outlook. Ordinarily, a book is a reflection of the scholarly output of its writer within the time and space context. As a humble researcher and health educationist, I must acknowledge any effort and goodwill that adds to the successful publication of this work and indeed my literary endeavour in general. I was greatly inspired and motivated by the generous comments, support and encouragement received from many giants during the first public presentation of this work.

Their Excellencies; General Yakubu Gowon, Admiral Mike Okhai Akhigbe and Dr Joseph Wayas, who graciously attended the occasion, provided the tripod upon which the public presentation of the book was successfully anchored. I am equally grateful to Their Royal Highnesses; His Eminence the Sultan of Sokoto, Alhaji Sa'ad Abubakar III, Alhaji Samaila Mera (Emir of Argungu) and Major General Sani Sami (Emir of Zuru) for their fatherly blessings and noble representations. I owe special gratitude to His Royal Highness, Dr Haliru Yahaya, the Emir of Shonga (Kwara State) for delivering the keynote speech that became the galvanizing fore for scholarly discourse. In the same vein, I acknowledged other dignitaries particularly; Alhaji M.D. Yusuf, Justice Umaru Abdullahi, Justice Aboki, Prof. Dora

Akunyili, General A.B. Dambazau, Prof. Abdul Aguye, Prof. H.G Sharubutu and the representatives of the Governor of Kebbi State and the Chief of the Naval Staff. My profound thanks are due to Professor Temitope Alonge (Chief Medical Director, University College Hospital Ibadan) and Prof Habib Galadanci (formerly Director Institute of Virology, Abuja) for their scholarly review and invaluable inputs as book reviewers.

First and foremost, my thanks and gratitude is due to God Almighty without whose help nothing can ever be accomplished. I am thankful to all and anyone He has used towards the success of this publication. It is not possible to mention all, but I will apologetically mention a few.

I must begin with the Chief of the Naval Staff, Vice Admiral Dele Ezeoba for his gracious permission to publish my works and their presentation to the public. The CNS, as the Commanding Officer of Nigerian Navy Ship ARADU when I was the Medical Officer publication onboard, was always a source of inspiration for research and intellectual profundity. I am similarly grateful to the Flag Officer Commanding Naval Training Command Rear Admiral I.A. Ajuonu for the order he gave to the CABO to "encourage the young man" which turned out to be a generous package. I must acknowledge the contributions of Rear Admiral A. Johnson, the Commandant Nigerian Naval College of Engineering towards the success of this publication.

I must express my special appreciation to Rear Admirals DJ. Boer, A. Shettima and B.M. Mshelia for their fatherly support and encouragement. I am thankful to Commander A Aminu, Command Accounts and Budget Officer (CABO), Naval Training Command for his moral and financial contributions towards the success of this and other publications. I must acknowledge the contributions of the following: Captains I.J Ahmed, EB Duke, S.S. Seidu, BM Idris, IA Shettima; Commanders Ngatuwa, ID Nuruddeen, Lieutenant Commander HON Asiboja, Lieutenants S.O.

Bada, Surgeon Sub Lieutenants B. Adamu and Basaru and my professional colleagues at the Naval Medical Centre Sapele.

Corporal Augustine Yahaya of the Nigerian Army deserves special mention for the typesetting, editorial work and cover design. I am no less thankful to my boys; AB Ketebu, Seamen Oloade, Aminu, Andrew, OS Omojofodun and Mr Desire Itidiare for their help in so many ways. Finally, I am indebted to my family for their abiding prayers and goodwill always. To all I say, *Meici Beacoup* (Thank you)!

> *"It is one of the beautiful compensations of this life that no man can sincerely help another without helping himself"*
> *– Ralph Waldo Emerson*

I am also thankful to Alhaji Abubakar Mudi Kangiwa (formerly the Accountant General, Kebbi State) for his fatherly role in my affairs and ample encouragement. I am deeply grateful to Malam Lawali Abubakar, Dr Mahmoud Garba, Alhaji Lawali Labbo (Magatakarda), Malam Aliyu Dodge, members of Dikko family especially Alhaji Aminu, Engr Yusuf, Malam Shehu Adamu, Aminu Bello Dange and my friends; Malam Sani, Abdullahi Sakibu and Usman Uzo *(the Wonderful Three)* for their loyal companionship and sacrifices at all times. I am also indebted to my colleagues in the Navy, particularly, Lieutenant Commanders A.A. Yabo, A.M. Idu, N. Lawali and G. A. Babalola for their support and encouragement.

In general, I commend all those whose support and cooperation positively influenced the successful outcome of this work.

Umar Faruk Adamu
Directorate of Medical Services
Nigerian Navy

Abbreviations

CAM	Complementary Alternative Medicine
GCP	Good Clinical Practice
CMC	Captain Medical Centre
GLP	Good Laboratory Practice
GMP	Good Manufacturing Practice
HFA	Health For All
MDCN	Medical and Dental Council of Nigeria
MRS	Medical Reception Station
NAFDAC	National Agency for Food and Drug Administration and Control
NICTAM	National Investigative Committee on Traditional and Alternative Medicine
NIPRD	National Institute for Pharmaceutical Research and Development
NMC	Naval Medical Centre
NUMHP	Nigerian Union of Medical Herbal Practitioners
OMP	Orthodox Medical Practitioner
PCN	Pharmaceutical Council of Nigeria
PHC	Primary Health Care
TBA	Traditional Birth Attendant
TM	Traditional Medicine
TMP	Traditional Medical Practitioner

Introduction

Medical practice today is a culmination of man's quest for health through the ages, which has been built up in various societies and at various times. In essence, the dichotomy between modern and traditional medicine is almost artificial. What is called modern medicine today was originally traditional. The history of medicine is therefore a review of accomplishments and errors, the evolution of man and human knowledge down the ages, and of the ever-changing concepts, goals and objectives of medicine in the course of time. This has proceeded by stages, with advances and halts; it has taken the wisdom of many peoples, and gleaned from their traditional cultures and later, from biological and natural sciences, and more recently, from social, behavioural and genetic sciences.

The battle between man and disease is indeed not a new one. In spite of the development from the earliest stage of superstition and witchcraft to the remarkable advances in modern era of rational chemotherapy and genetic manipulations, the fight has been more intense than ever before. The threat posed by certain major diseases has not lessened, in some cases it has actually increased. Life expectancy particularly in the developing countries is sadly on the decline, while death rates is unacceptably high on the rise. This situation or predicament is more pronounced in poorer countries where an interplay of poverty, hunger and ignorance stifle some of the gains recorded in modern medicine[1].With increasing recognition of the failure of existing health services to provide health care to all people and in all communities, alternative ideas and methods to provide health services have been considered and tried. As a result of these incongruities, traditional medicine is now attracting a renewed attention worldwide.

In Nigeria, for quite a long time, many medical scholars have advocated that attention should be given to traditional medicine as an alternative or complementary system of medicine for example, in the early 60's, Prof. Adeoye Lambo, saw the need to integrate some aspects of traditional medicine into the country's health care system.

Similarly in the 70's, Prof. Umaru Shehu (then) of Ahmadu Bello University, Zaria advocated the use of traditional healers in the cure of the mentally disturbed, and the use of traditional midwives in the rural areas where there is difficult access to modern health care machinery. Perhaps it was a response to such appeals, that the Federal Ministry of Health sent a fact-finding mission to India and China to study their systems of traditional medicine and relationship with orthodox practice. Again, about five years later, a National Committee on Traditional and Alternative Medicine (NICTAM) was set up to harness the resources in traditional medicine. In the global scene, following the famous Alma-Ata Declaration of 1978 and its declared target of "Health for All", the World Health Organisation (WHO) saw the need to incorporate traditional medicine into its programme.

Despite the growing interest in traditional medicine as an integral part of health care delivery, the bulk of it still remains unofficial, crude and sometimes, a harmful part of health care system in Nigeria. This observation may account for the contempt and distrust existing between the traditional healers and their orthodox counterparts, with each group claiming supremacy and relevance over the other. Heaps of criticisms and arguments have been advanced to discredit one system or the other. While this war was on going, the government seems to have maintained an attitude of "leave them alone" towards some practitioners of traditional medicine. However, this situation does not help matters, because as long as modern medicine continues to remain costly, heavily bureaucratised and elitist-oriented, majority of the populace will continue trooping to traditional clinics and healing homes in order to find succour and solace in the hands of the uncurbed and poorly-regulated traditional healers.

The way things are going on now is rather an unfortunate development. There is no need to allow the two systems to operate along two opposing and confrontational lines. Needless to say that despite the fact that both medical systems have merits and demerits, yet the exact relationship between them is uncertain. At different times, it may be complementary, supplementary, competitive, or even contradictory. What is clear, however, is that given the existing situation, some form of regulation between the two systems is necessary in maintaining vertical or parallel services. However, whether this should take the form of separation or integration is still a matter of debate and intellectual discussion.

This book advances certain questions and raises them to the level of theoretical debate and intellectual discourse. The questions are:

- What constitutes traditional or modern medicine?
- What are the criticisms against them and how are they refuted?

- How do you identify the beneficial, neutral, harmless and harmful aspects of the practice of indigenous medicine?

- What aspects of these, should or should not be integrated?

- What are the modifications the orthodox practitioner has to make? What are the problems and prospects of integration?

This book may not have adequate answers for all these questions, nor does it attempt to do so. However, its aim is to hopefully stimulate thought-provoking discourse, so as to promote better understanding of the two systems. At the end, individuals, professional bodies and governments can be better placed to make appropriate choices for improved health care delivery and human progress.

Definitions of Terms and Terminologies

(a) **Traditional medicine** is the sum total of the knowledge, skills, and practices based on the theories, beliefs, and experiences indigenous to different cultures, whether explicable or not, used in the maintenance of health as well as in the prevention, diagnosis, improvement or treatment of physical and mental illnesses. In other words, traditional medicine comprises therapeutic practices that have been in existence, often for hundreds of years, before the development and spread of modern scientific medicine. These practices are still in use today.

(b) **Complementary alternative medicine** is a term used in some developing countries where the dominant health care system is based on allopathic medicine, or where traditional medicine has not been incorporated into the national health care system. Other names used for traditional medicine are: unofficial, unorthodox, pre-scientific, fringe, indigenous, ancient, folk and ethno medicine.[2]

(c) **Modern medicine** refers to the dominant health system of medicine officially approved, patronised, funded and provided by the government to take care of the health of the people. Other names for modern medicine are: allopathic, orthodox, scientific, classical, conventional and Western.

(d) **Pharmaceutical product** refers to "any product intended for human use or veterinary product administered to food-producing animals, presented in its finished dosage form or as a starting material or use in such a dosage form that is subject to control by pharmaceutical legislation in both the exporting state and the importing state". By this definition, herbal medicines are pharmaceutical products.

(e) A World Health Organisation Scientific Group has defined a **drug** as "any substance or product that is used or intended to be used to modify or explore physiological systems or pathological states for the benefit of the recipient". In other words, a drug is simply "any substance that brings about a change in biologic function through its chemical actions". This definition is not restrictive, that is, it does not distinguish whether a drug is synthetic or natural, or whether it is in processed form or it exists in local herbage. A drug, therefore, is a single chemical substance that forms the active ingredient of a medicine whereas a medicine is a substance or mixture of substances used in restoring or preserving health. Therefore, a medicine may contain many other substances to deliver the drug in a stable form, acceptable and convenient to the patient. The terms (drug and medicine) are sometimes used more or less interchangeably.

(f) **A medicinal plant** is any plant which, in one or more of its organs, contain substances that can be used for therapeutic purposes or which are precursors for the synthesis of useful drugs. The term concoction in the pharmaceutical sense means a preparation made usually from many ingredients, whereas decoction is the aqueous extract of a plant preparation or mixture.

(g) The World Heath Organisation also defines **herbal medicines** as "finished, labeled medicinal products that contain as active ingredients, aerial or underground parts of plants or other plant materials, or combinations thereof, whether in the crude state or as plant preparations". Another term used is phytomedicine. They include herbs, herbal materials, herbal preparations and finished herbal products that contain as active ingredients parts of plants, or other plant materials, or combinations. Traditional use of herbal medicines refers to the long historical use of these medicines. Their use is well established and widely acknowledged to be safe and effective, and may be accepted by national authorities.

- *herbs* include crude plant material such as leaves, flowers, fruits, seeds, stems, woods, barks, roots, rhizomes or other plant parts, which may be entire, fragmented or powdered.

- *herbal materials* include, in addition to herbs, fresh juices, gums, fixed oils, essential oils, resins and dry powders of herbs. In some countries, these materials may be processed by various local procedures, such as steaming, roasting, or stir-baking with honey, alcoholic beverages or other materials.

- *herbal preparations* are the basis for finished herbal products and may include comminuted or powdered herbal materials, or extracts, tinctures and fatty oils of herbal materials. They are produced by extraction, fractionation, purification, concentration, or other physical or biological processes. They also include preparations made by steeping or heating herbal materials in alcoholic beverages and/or honey, or in other materials.

- *finished herbal products* consist of herbal preparations made from one or more herbs. If more than one herb is used, the term mixture herbal products can also be used; Finished herbal products and mixture herbal products may contain excipients in addition to the active ingredients. However, finished products or mixture products to which chemically defined active substances have been added, including synthetic compounds and/or isolated constituents from herbal materials, are not considered to be herbal.

(h) **Therapeutic activity** refers to the successful prevention, diagnosis and treatment of physical and mental illnesses; improvement of symptoms of illnesses; as well as beneficial alteration or regulation of the physical and mental status of the body. Active ingredients refer to ingredients of herbal medicines with therapeutic activity. In herbal medicines where the active ingredients have been identified, the preparation of these medicines should be standardised to contain a defined amount of the active ingredients, if adequate analytical methods are available. In cases where it is not possible to identify the active ingredients, the whole herbal medicine may be considered as one active ingredient.

(i) The term **traditional medical practitioners** comprise a variety of practitioners of traditional medicine ranging from spiritualists, traditional birth attendants, bonesetters, magicians and those dealing with herbs (herbalists). A traditional medical practitioner can be described as 'a person who is recognised by the community in which he lives as competent to provide health care by using vegetable, animal and mineral substances, and certain other methods'. These methods are based on social, cultural, and religious background as well as on the knowledge, attitudes, and beliefs that are prevalent in the community regarding physical, mental and social well-being and the causes of disease and disability. Other terms used for traditional medical practitioner are traditional healer, native doctor, indigenous practitioner, traditional health practitioner, etc.

(j) An **orthodox medical practitioner** refers to a practitioner who uses modern, conventional or scientific means and methods in the maintenance, promotion, or restoration of health and prevention of diseases. The term *likita* commonly used by the Hausa-speaking people of Northern Nigeria, is an exclusive reserve of the orthodox medical practitioner. *Boka* refers to the herbalist, who is regarded as the mainstream of traditional medical practice, analogous to the way the term *physician* becomes applicable synonymously to any orthodox medical practitioner.

(k) **Integration** in this context refers to the incorporation or rehabilitation of traditional healers into the officially recognised health care system of a country and training of health practitioners to know something about both systems of medicine. On the other hand, co-recognition refers to the legal recognition of traditional medicine as an independent official method of health care and its practice side by side with modern medicine, otherwise called *parallel* medical services.

Historical Overview

The longer you can look back, the further you can look forward. For those who fail to read history are destined to suffer the repetition of its mistakes – Winston Churchill

It has been said that medicine was conceived in sympathy, and born out of necessity; and that the first doctor was the first man; and the first woman, the first nurse. This may be true in view of the fact that the prehistoric man, motivated by feelings of sympathy and kindness, was always at the behest of his relations and neighbours, trying to provide relief in times of sickness and suffering.

From time immemorial, man has been interested in trying to curb, control or contain disease. Thus, the 'medicine-man', the priest, the herbalist and the magician, all undertook in various ways to cure man's disease and bring relief to the sick. In an almost complete absence of scientific medical knowledge, it would be unfair to say that the early (traditional) medical practitioners contributed nothing to the alleviation of man's suffering and fight against disease, both known and unknown.

In reality, our current medical knowledge has been derived to a very great degree, from the cumulative experience of man as he wades through the annals of history right from primitive to present times. In other words, modern medicine is what it is today because it has drawn richly from the traditional cultures of several peoples and societies, at different periods of time developing stage by stage. Thus, modern medicine is built on the best of the past.

Primitive Medicine

In ancient times, health and illness were interpreted in cosmological and anthropological perspectives. Since his knowledge was limited, the primitive man attributed disease, and in fact all human suffering and other calamities, to the wrath of gods, the invasion of body by malevolent demons, who were believed to project an alien spirit, a stone, or a worm into the body of the unsuspecting patient. This concept of disease was known as the "supernatural theory of disease". As a logical sequence, the medicine he practised consisted in appeasing gods by prayers, incantations, rituals, and sacrifices, driving out evil spirits from the human body by witchcraft and other crude means, and the use of charms and amulets as a means of protection against their influences or effects.

Later on, another dimension was added to this spiritualism; the empirical administration of herbs and animal parts propelled by the urge to "do something". It is thus obvious that medicine in the prehistoric times (about 5000 BC) was the result of the interplay between superstitions, religion, magic, witchcraft and empiricism.

Indian Medicine

The Indian medicine or *Ayurveda,* which by definition means 'knowledge of life', show a rather advanced knowledge of sanitation, water supply and engineering. Of significance in *Ayurvedic* medicine is the *"tridosha* theory of disease". The *doshas* or humours are *vata* (wind), *pitta* (gall) and *kapha* (mucus). Disease was explained as a disturbance in the equilibrium of the three humours; and when these were in perfect balance and harmony, a person is said to be healthy. This theory of disease is strikingly similar to the "theory of four humours" in Greek medicine.

Medical historians admit that, there was free exchange of thoughts and experiences between the Hindu, Arab, Persian, Greek and Jewish scholars. While it can be said that *Ayurveda* has some useful remedies, the religious orthodoxy which prohibited the study of anatomy using cadavers (dead human bodies) was partly responsible for the stagnation of this system of medicine.

The practices of *Ayuverda,* or vedantic medicine, (1500-1000 BC) are described in the works of two later physicians, Charaka and Susruta. Susruta gave recognisable description of malaria, tuberculosis, and diabetes. He also wrote about Indian hemp *(Cannabis sativa)* and henbane *(Hyoscyamus niger)* for inducing anaesthesia, and included specific antidotes and highly skilled treatments for the bites of venomous snakes. An ancient Hindu drug derived from the root of the Indian hemp plant was the source of the first modern tranquilliser. In the field of operative surgery, the Indians are acknowledged to have attained the highest skill in all antiquity. They were probably the first to perform successful skin grafting and plastic surgery for the nose.

The golden age of Indian medicine was between 800 BC and 600 AD. Other indigenous systems of Indian medicine include homeopathy and *Unani-Tibb.* Unani-Tibb was introduced into India by the Muslim rulers about the 10th century AD. It enjoyed state support under successive rulers in India, till the advent of the British in the 18th century. The Indian systems of medicine (including Unani-Tibb and homeopathy) are very much alive in India even today. In fact, they have become part of Indian culture, and continue to be an important source of medical service to the rural population.

Chinese Medicine

Chinese medicine claims to be the world's first organised body of medical knowledge dating back to about 2500 BC. It is based on two principles – the *yang* (an active masculine principle) and the *yin* (a negative feminine principle). The balance of these two opposing forces meant good health. Hygiene, dietetics, hydrotherapy, massage, and drugs were all used by the Chinese physicians.

The Chinese up till today have great faith in their heritage in traditional medicine, which is fully integrated with modern medicine. Their system of medicine produces great advances in preventive medicine. To the Chinese, "the great doctor is one who treats not someone who is already ill but someone not yet ill". The Chinese system of "barefoot doctors" and acupuncture has attracted worldwide attention in recent years.

Egyptian Medicine

Egyptian medicine was far from primitive because Egypt had one of the oldest civilisations. They believed that disease was due to absorption from the intestine of harmful substances which gave rise to putrefaction of blood and formation of pus. They believed that the pulse was "the speech of the heart". Diseases were treated with cathartics, enema, bloodletting and a wide range of drugs. In the realm of public health also, the Egyptians excelled. They built planned cities, public baths and underground drain which even the modem might envy.

The best-known medical manuscripts belonging to the Egyptian times are the Edwin Smiths' *Papyrus* (1600 BC), the oldest treatise on surgery, and the Ebers' *Papyrus* (1150 BC). The former, containing a description of forty-eight cases and written almost in modern style, accurately describes partial paralysis following injury to the head (cerebral lesions), while the latter contains a unique record of some 800 prescriptions based on some 7000 drugs. Although Egyptians practised embalming, their anatomical knowledge remained at low level; as a result they attempted only minor surgical procedures. Egyptian medicine occupied a dominant place in the ancient world for many centuries before it was replaced by Greek medicine.

Mesopotamian Medicine

Contemporary with ancient Egyptian civilisation was the ancient civilisation of Mesopotamia; an area which lies between the Tigris and Euphrates rivers (parts of what constitute Middle East particularly Iraq). The basic concepts of medicine at the time were religiously taught and practised by *herb doctors, knife doctors* and *spell doctors* - a classification that roughly parallels our own internists, surgeons and psychiatrists. Of particular importance was the famous code of Hammurabi, after a great king of Babylon, who lived around 2000 BC. The code regulated medical practice and laid down penalties for harmful therapy and quackery, even though the basis of medicine at the time was devoid of any known scientific foundation.

Hebrew Medicine

Hebrew medicine derived much from contact with Mesopotamian medicine during the Assyrian and Babylonian captivities. Disease was considered evidence of the wrath of God. The priesthood acquired the responsibility for compiling hygienic regulations, and the status of the midwife as an assistant in childbirth was clearly defined. Although the Old Testament contains a few references to diseases caused by the intrusion of spirits, the tone of biblical medicine is modern in its marked emphasis on preventing disease. The Book of Leviticus includes precise instructions on such varied subjects as feminine hygiene, segregation of the sick, and disinfection of materials capable of harbouring and transmitting germs. Although circumcision is the only surgical procedure clearly described, fractures were treated with the roller bandage, and wounds were dressed with oil, wine, and balsam. The leprosy (Hansen's disease) so frequently mentioned in the Bible is now believed to have embraced many skin diseases, including psoriasis.

Greek Medicine

After the Egyptian medicine, next came the Greek medicine whose classic period ranged from 460 to 136 BC. Greeks were the pioneers of modern medicine. It was to their credit that they gave a new direction to medical thought. They rejected the 'supernatural theory of diseases' and brought the "theory of the four humours" - *phlegm, yellow bile, blood* and *black bile*. The theory postulated that health prevailed when the four humours were in equilibrium and that disease result when the balance is disturbed. The human body was assumed to have powers of restoration of equilibrium (a valid theory even today), and it was the physician's primary role to assist in this healing process.

By separating magic and superstition from medicine and based their practice on clinical history, physical examination and experience of various cases, the Greek physicians laid the foundation of scientific medicine in 5th century BC. By far, the greatest physician in Greek medicine was Hippocrates (460 - 370 BC) who is often called the "Father of Medicine". He challenged the tradition of magic and superstition in medicine and initiated a new radical approach - the application of clinical and rational methods in medicine. He studied and classified diseases based on observation and reasoning. His famous oath, the "Hippocratic Oath" has become the cornerstone of medical ethics[3] and sets a high moral standard for the medical profession and demands absolute integrity. He will always be remembered as the man who changed the destiny of medicine by separating it from magic and raising it to the status of a Science.

Roman Medicine

The glorious Greek civilisation fell into decay and by the 1st century BC, the centre of civilisation had shifted to Rome. The Romans borrowed their medicine largely from the Greeks whom they had conquered, but they were a more practical-minded people than the Greeks. Public health was born in Rome with the development of public baths, sewers and aqueducts through which they brought water and drained marshes to combat malaria. They established hospitals for the sick. An outstanding figure among Roman medical teachers was Galen (130- 205 AD), whose writings influenced both Arab and European medicine for centuries.

Medicine in the Middle Ages

The period between 500 and 1500 AD is generally known as the 'Middle Ages'. With the fall of the Roman Empire, medical knowledge stagnated for a while. Europe was ravaged by diseases and pestilence such as plague, small pox, leprosy and tuberculosis. As a result of the influence of Christianity, rejection of the body and glorification of the spirit became the accepted pattern of behaviour. It was regarded as immoral to see one's body; consequently dissection of the human body was prohibited. The progress made by medicine was stifled and its practice reverted back to primitive methods dominated by superstition and dogma. Consequently, there was no progress of medicine. The period was therefore called the "Dark Ages of Medicine".

This period also witnessed the persecution of practitioners of an empirical folk medicine that was in opposition to the professional physicians. This persecution of alleged witches and spiritualists may have had its origin in the efforts of the church to stamp out the remnants of paganism among the people. However, with time the persecution was revived, intensified and shifted to professional physicians who were condemned for either contradicting Holy Scriptures or "attributing too much to nature, casting aside the Author of nature". Hence, the saying "Where there are three physicians, there are two atheists" became a common proverb in Europe. The church then, sternly forbade scientific explorations and theories that seems to threaten its authority and dogma, just as it forbade teaching certain discoveries in universities and centres of learning

Subsequently, the idea that too bold an inquiry into the ways of nature was dangerous became a part of religious thinking. For instance, physicians were looked at suspiciously, especially if they were followers of Avicenna (lbn Sina) and Averroes (lbn Rushd), the famous Islamic philosophers and medical authorities. Although medicine was in a primitive state, the very fact that these men regarded disease as something other than the possession by demons or inflictions from God made them somewhat dangerous characters at the time.

This era represent the period when science was struggling to emerge from magic and superstition and re-establish itself. However, the warfare (between science and the church) continued into the 19th century, which however witnessed the revolutionalisation of medical knowledge.

Arab Medicine

In the 7th century, a vast portion of the Eastern world was overrun by Arab conquerors. Thus when Europe was passing through the Dark Ages, the Arabs took over the leadership of civilisation. Utilising the body of knowledge inherited from previous civilisations particularly the Greek, they developed their own system of medicine known as the *Unani- Tibb* system of medicine'.

They founded schools of medicine and hospitals in Baghdad, Damascus, Cairo, Cordoba and other Muslim capitals. Parallel to the Islamic political expansion, Islamic medicine also, came to be practised across a vast geographical area, stretching from; India, via North Africa, to Spain, and spanning from the middle of the 8th to the middle of the 17th centuries. The most famous Islamic physician is Abu Ali Ibn Sina (980-1037), Latinised as Avicenna. He composed several small writings dealing with diverse medical topics such as sexual hygiene, cardiac drugs, bloodletting, diagnosis according to respiration and pulse, intermittent fevers, and diabetes. However, he is universally recognised as the author of the *Canon of Medicine,* a massive encyclopedia embracing all the theoretical principles of the medical profession, composed over a lengthy period of time. Due to its exhaustive systematisation of medical knowledge, it became an authoritative stock of medical information, both as a textbook for students of medicine and as a reference book for medical practitioners. This work was the most influential Arabic medical text in European medical schools and universities. Ibn Sina, an intellectual prodigy, was responsible for elevating 'Islamic medicine' to its zenith in the middle ages.

Another leader in Arabic medicine was Ibn Razi (also known as Rhazes). Rhazes was a director of a large hospital in Baghdad as well as a court physician. He was noted for his keen observation and inventiveness. He was the first to observe pupillary reaction to light, to use mercurial purgatives, and to publish the first known book on children's diseases - smallpox and measles.

The greatest contribution of Arabs in general, was in the field of pharmacology. They introduced a large number of drugs, herbs and chemical compounds and also invented the art of writing prescription, and introduced the use of a wide range of substances such as oils, poultices, plasters, powders, alcoholates and aromatic waters in medical practice. The words *drug, alcohol, syrup, alkali, tartar* and *sugar* are all Arabian. The golden age of Arabic medicine was between 810-1310 AD.

The Birth of Modern Medicine

The revival of medicine encompasses the period from 1400 -1600 AD. It was an age of individual scientific endeavour, when "Europe stretched her limbs after a sleep of a thousand years in a bed of darkness". This period witnessed many discoveries. Fracustorius (1483-1553) enunciated the "theory of contagion" - that diseases can be transmitted from one person to another. Andreas Vasalius (1514 -1564) raised the study of anatomy to a science. The 17th and 18th centuries were full of even more exciting discoveries for example, Harvey's discovery of the circulation of blood (1628), Leeuwenhoek's microscope (1670) and Jenners' vaccination against small pox (1796).

For long, man was groping in darkness about the causation of disease. Several theories were advanced from time to time to explain disease causation such as the supernatural theory of disease, the theory of our humours by Greeks, the theory of contagion, the theory of spontaneous generation, and so on. It was not until 1860, when Louis Pasteur (1822-1895) demonstrated the presence of bacteria in air, and Robert Koch (1843-1910) showed that bacteria caused anthrax, that the "germ theory of disease" was advanced. Thereafter, microbe after microbe was discovered in quick succession.

Immediately after the discovery of microbial organisms, another profound revolution took place. That was the discovery of anti-microbial agents like penicillin and development of vaccines. This was followed by the development of allopathic medicine-treatment of disease by the use of a drug, which produces reaction that itself neutralises the disease. This was the era of drugs being used as 'magic bullets'.

After 1900, medicine moved faster towards specialisation and a rational, scientific approach to disease. The pattern of disease began to change, with the control of infectious diseases such as tuberculosis, pneumonia, leprosy, particularly in the developed world. Then came the emergence of the so-called modern diseases-hypertension, mental illnesses, cancer, etc. These diseases could not be explained on the basis of the "germ theory of disease", nor treated with "magic bullets".

The realisation began to dawn on the scientists that, there are other factors in the aetiology of diseases namely social, economic, genetic, environmental and psychological which are equally important. Most of these factors are linked to man's lifestyle, behaviour and environment. Thus, the germ theory of disease gave rise to a new concept of disease - "multi-factorial causation". This concept laid an increased emphasis on the unity of man's nature. It recognises more and more that a patient need not be regarded as an interesting case of this, that or the other but a holistic and total entity. And that the causes of much physical illnesses and mental disturbances are to be found in the deep and intimate relationship of the physical, mental, spiritual and social dimensions of life.

Medicine today has moved much more rapidly from the organism to organ, and from the organ to the cells, and from the cell to the molecular level. The discovery of the biological role of nucleic acids, the uncovering of the genetic code and its role in regulating life processes are marvelous discoveries in recent years. Medicine has acquired a vast body of knowledge and has become highly sophisticated and technical. It has acquired new capabilities to modify and perhaps control the capacities and activities of mankind by direct intervention into and manipulation of their bodies and minds, through many revolutionary methods. Such methods include genetic counseling and engineering, prenatal diagnosis of sex and diseases, *invitro* fertilisation, the prospect of cloning (the asexual production of unlimited number of genetically identical individual from a single parent), organ transplantation and the use of artificial kidney machine, the development of an artificial heart, the practice of neuro-surgery, the use of life support machines, etc. This is how medicine has evolved down the centuries, and it will continue to evolve so long as man's quest for better health continues.

Truly, Western medicine was in the beginning little better than the different indigenous systems of medicine like Arabic, Hellenic (Greek), *Ayuverdic* or Chinese. For instance, the *London Pharmacopoeia* of the seventeenth century had medicines including the "blood of the bat and badger, skulls of male factors, eel grease, viper's flesh, and wood lice." An 18th century French dictionary of drugs contains a prescription of *"fresh urine two or three glasses every morning is good for gout, hysteria and obstruction; excreta of man can be applied to anthrax, hysteria, and quinsies."*

Today, its claims to be counted *modern* is due to several advantages that it enjoyed in the course of its development. These advantages are its association with other modern sciences, its intellectual tradition of free inquiry and precise observation, its spirit of humanism and its status as an enlightened liberal profession. This is how medicine has evolved down the centuries. Thus, Western medicine, which is today modern medicine, is not only international, but also multiracial.

However, modern medicine will not have completed its mission until its main spirit and outlook permeate every practitioner of it:

• That medicine is a humane art enriched by years of sacrifices, that it deals kindly with all,

• That it is a wise art that addresses the whole dimension of life and living experience, and

• Finally, that character counts far more than other virtues among its practitioners.

Current Scenario

'Failure of Success'

Despite the spectacular achievements of modern medicine, the improvements in health-status indicators (such as life expectancy and infant mortality) of people in the developed world owe more to an improved availability of food, and improving economic development, public health, and sanitation measures, than to conventional medicine *per se.* In the light of this, as well as because of the burgeoning costs of modern medicine, the World Health Organisation (WHO) stresses and promotes the role of public-health measures (including preventive and community-based approaches, improved food supply, sanitation, and education) along with affordable medicine using appropriate technology, to achieve health for large populations of the developing world in a reasonable span of time.

Today, modern medicine has developed more rapidly in several areas of specialisations thereby fragmenting health care delivery into too great a degree. It is no longer solely an art and science for the diagnosis and treatment of diseases. It is also the science for the prevention of disease and the promotion of health. The scope of medicine has expanded during the last few decades to include not only the health of individuals, but those of communities as well.

Specialisation and Microspecialisation

In reviewing the history of medicine during the past one hundred years, it would be appreciated that tremendous growth of specialisation has taken place in response to advances in medical technology due to changes in the nature and distribution of health and disease pattern in the community, and to the changing emphasis placed by society upon age and sex groups. Some specialties have emerged, based on clearly defined skills such as surgery, radiology, and anaesthesia; some based on parts of the body such as ENT (ear-nose and throat! otorhinolaryngology), ophthalmology, cardiology, gynaecology; and some based on particular age or sex groups such as paediatrics, geriatrics and obstetrics. Again within each specialty, there has been a growth of sub-specialties, for example, neonatology, perinatology, paediatric cardiology, paediatric neurology and paediatric surgery – all in paediatrics.

Specialisation has no doubt raised the standards of medical care but it has escalated the cost of medical care and placed specialist medical care beyond the means of an average citizen, without outside aid or charity. It has infringed upon the basic tenets of socialism (i.e. the greatest good to the greatest number) and paved the way to varying degrees of social control over medicine. Specialisation has also contributed to the decline of general practice and the isolation of medical practitioners at the periphery of the medical care system.

Criticisms

From the foregoing, it is glaring that modern medicine has entered a new evolutionary stage with the promise of continued improvement in medical capabilities to preserve life, and solve problems of diseases and medical disorders. Yet, today a great skepticism surrounds medical care. Like so many other institutions in contemporary society, medicine as practised today, has come under heavy fire and flak. It has begun to be questioned and criticised disparagingly. Some critics have even described modern medicine as a threat to health. Their arguments have been based on certain facts such as:

(a) With increased medical costs has not come increased benefits in terms of health;

(b) Despite the spectacular advances in medicine, the threat posed by certain major diseases such as malaria, tuberculosis and leprosy, either has not lessened or has actually increased;

(c) Life expectancy has remained low and infant and maternal mortality rates high in many developing countries;

(d) Significant improvement in longevity had been achieved through improved food supplies and sanitation long before the advent of modern drugs and high technology; and

(e) Lack of equity in the distribution of health services resulting in limited access to health care for large segments of the world's population.

The above observations unfold the glaring contrasts in the picture of health in developed and developing countries. High technology medicine seems to be getting out of hand and leading health systems in the wrong direction, that is, away from the health promotion for the many and towards expensive treatment for the few. For example, most people in the developed countries, and the elite of the developing countries, enjoy all the determinants of good health - adequate income, nutrition, education, sanitation, safe drinking water and comprehensive health care. In contrast, only ten to twenty per cent of the populations in developing countries enjoy ready access to health services of any kind.

Not only is there an increasing concern about the cost and allocation of health resources, but the efficacy of modern medicine is fundamentally questioned from various points of view. It has given rise to the notion that limits had been reached on the health impact of medical care and research. This has been labeled as a "failure of success".

Disparity in Health Care Services

In Africa, due to the poverty and infrastructural insufficiency at all levels, the health care coverage is limited. A death claim 60-250 of every 1000 live births within the first year of life and life expectancy is 30% lower than in the developed countries. No wonder John Bryant in the introduction to his book, *Health and the Developing World* presented a gloomy picture of the real situation, saying:

Large numbers of the world's population, perhaps more than half, have no access to health care at all, and for many of the rest the care they receive does not answer the problems they have.

This situation has generated a feeling that medicine was not rendering its full service to humanity. As the cost of medical care increased; two kinds of medical care came into existence - one for the rich and the other for the poor. The gap was bridged to a small extent by charitable and voluntary organizations/agencies providing free medical care to the poor.

As a result of this disparity, which awkwardly manifests as social injustice, the global conscience was stirred leading to a new awakening that the health gap between rich and poor within countries and between countries should be narrowed and ultimately eliminated, so that the benefits of modern medicine are made available to all people. It is conceded that the neglected 80% of the world's population too have an equal claim to health care, protection from the killer diseases of childhood, primary health care for mothers and children, treatment for those ills that mankind has long ago learnt to control, if not cure, and protection from preventable diseases.

Primary Health Care and Traditional Medicine

With increasing recognition of the failure of existing health services to provide health care to all people and in all communities, alternative ideas and methods to provide health services have been considered and tried. In September 1978, at Alma-Ata in the former USSR, a joint WHO-UNICEF international conference attended by representatives of the governments of 134 countries and many voluntary organisations, called for a revolutionary approach to health care, and a declaration was made, ever since, known as the Alma-Ata Declaration.

The members of the WHO pledged themselves to an ambitious target to provide health for all by the year 2000, and proclaimed primary health care (PHC) as a way of achieving that goal. That is attainment of a level of health that will permit all peoples of the world "to lead a socially and economically productive life". *Health-for-all* means that, health is to be brought within the reach of every one-in a given community. It does not mean, or guarantee that, everyone must be free from ill-health or sickness at any specific period. Rather, it implies the removal of obstacles to health, that is to say, the elimination of malnutrition, ignorance, disease, contaminated water supply, unhygienic housing, etc. Though that utopian ambition has not been reached, PHC still remains the most effective tool of achieving the health-for-all target goals[5]. The PHC lays emphasis on preventive and simple health care adapted to local needs and resources.

The practice of PHC involves a good deal of "de-professionalisation" of medicine. It implies that health care delivery, in spite of its unique importance, must not be left in the hands of the professionals alone. Laymen have to come to play a prominent role in the health care delivery process. While the medical doctor still holds his unique position in the field of health care in general, the participation by a new cadre of health workers (for example; community health workers, traditional birth attendants, other practitioners of traditional medicine, social workers) with relatively little training and support have been considered and tried to provide or promote health care services. They now comprise part of the "health team".

In order to meet the growing challenges in health care services, the WHO has considered the integration of some aspect of traditional medicine in organised health care delivery. It has also provided policy guidelines for member states to help develop the potential for TM as a source of health care. While China, the Democratic People's Republic of Korea, the Republic of Korea and Vietnam have fully integrated TM into their health care systems, many countries are yet to collect and standardised evidence on this type of health care. However, WHO has launched its first ever comprehensive traditional medicine strategy in 2002. The strategy is designed to assist countries to:

- develop national policies on the evaluation and regulation of TMICAM practices;
- create a stronger evidence base on the safety, efficacy and quality of the TMICAM products and practices;
- ensure availability of TMICAM including essential herbal medicines;
- promote therapeutically sound use of TMICAM by providers and consumers; and
- document traditional medicines and remedies.

At present, WHO is supporting clinical studies on antimalarials in three African countries; the studies are revealing good potential for herbal antimalarials. Other collaboration is taking place with Burkina Faso, Democratic Republic of Congo, Ghana, Mali, Nigeria, Kenya, Uganda and Zimbabwe in the-research and evaluation of herbal treatments for HIV/AIDS, malaria, sickle cell disease and diabetes mellitus.

The potential of these studies are promising for example, the Chinese herbal remedy *Artemisia annua,* used in China for almost 2000 years has been found to be effective against resistant malaria and could create a breakthrough in preventing almost one million deaths annually, most of them children, from severe malaria. In South Africa, the medical research council is conducting studies on the efficacy of the plant *sutherlandia microphylla* in treating AIDS patients.

Traditionally used as tonic, this plant may increase energy, appetite and body mass in people living with HIV.

Increasing Use and Popularity

As a result of these efforts and several other factors, TM has maintained its popularity in all regions of the developing world and its use is rapidly spreading in industrialised countries. In China, traditional herbal preparations account for 30% - 50 % of the total medical consumption. In Ghana, Mali and Nigeria, the first line of treatment for 60% of children with high fever resulting from malaria is the use of herbal medicines at home. In several African countries, traditional birth attendants assist in the majority of births.

In Europe, North America and other industrialised regions, over 50% of the population have used complementary or alternative medicine at least once. In Canada, the percentage of such people is higher (about 70%). In Germany, 90% of the populations have used a natural remedy at some point in their life. Between 1995 and 2000, the number of orthodox practitioners who had undergone special training in natural remedy medicine has almost doubled to 10,800. While in the United States, 158 million of the adult population use complementary medicines and according to the USA Commission for Alternative and Complementary Medicine, US$17 billion was spent on traditional remedies in the year 2000. The global market for herbal medicines currently stands at over US$60 billion annually and is growing steadily.

Generally, the world's poorest countries are most in need of inexpensive, effective and treatment for diseases. WHO estimate that one-third of the world's population still lacks regular access to essential drugs; and that in the poorest parts of Africa and Asia, this figure rises to over 50%. In these regions, some form of traditional medicine is often a more widely available and affordable source of health care. Concerns about the adverse effects of chemical medicines, a desire for natural products and great public access to health information continue to fuel the increased use and attention paid to traditional medicines.

Further Challenges

Given the considerable regional diversity in the use of TM and appreciation of its role as an important source of health ,care particularly in developing countries, certain reservations must be made known. Firstly, it must be noted that unregulated or inappropriate use of traditional medicines and practices can have negative or dangerous effects. A growing number of reports document the sometimes fatal or adverse effects of misuse of traditional therapies and use of therapies for which information on safety is lacking. For instance, the herb *Ma Huang (Ephedra)* is traditionally used in China to treat respiratory congestion. In the US, the herb was marketed as dietary and its overdosage led to at least a dozen deaths, heart attacks and strokes. In Belgium, about 70 people had their kidney damaged irreversibly after taking a herbal preparation made from the wrong species of plant as slimming treatment.

In Nigeria, several cases abound, though not officially documented, of people suffering from a worsening medical condition consequent upon use of supplementary traditional products as substitute for definitive treatment of their ailments. The result has often times been fatal and catastrophic.

In addition to patient safety, there is the risk that uncontrolled use of a raw material for herbal medicines may lead to the extinction of the endangered species and the destruction of the natural habitats and resources. Another related issue is that at present, the requirements for protection provided under national and international standards for patent laws are inadequate to protect traditional knowledge and biodiversity. Preservation and protection of TM knowledge is essential to ensure access to traditional forms of health care and respects for those who hold TM knowledge.

A lot of difficulties are encountered in the scientific evaluation of TM products such as herbal medicines. This is because herbal" medicine quality is influenced by several factors, such as when and where the raw materials were collected, and accuracy of plant identification. Nevertheless, many TM practices and products have been used for considerable period of time. And some scientific evidence points to promising potential. Thus identification of safe and effective TM therapies must be made in order to provide a sound basis for efforts to promote TM. The focus should be on treatment for diseases which represent the greatest burden for poor populations, that is, for malaria and HIV/AIDS.

Of recent, the WHO Report of the Consultative Committee on AIDS and Traditional Medicine has advocated ways and means to expand the role of traditional health practitioner including traditional midwives, in the delivery of health services in African communities by actively involving them more in measures to prevent and control HIV infection and AIDS. If access to TM is to be increased to help improve health status, certain issues must be tackled.

Firstly, cooperation between TM providers and community health workers needs to be increased. In some countries, links between, for example, traditional birth attendants and primary health care providers are being strengthened. However, this is not the case in many other countries where these two types of health care provider work in isolation from one another, with the TM therapies being always sidelined from the mainstream conventional therapies. At the same time, some TM providers lack knowledge of PHC and perform practices that carry health risks and hazards. The challenge is to recognise and ensure that the health skills and knowledge of TM providers are optimised.

As of the year 2000, twenty-five countries have a national policy on traditional medicine. Such a policy provides a sound basis for defining the role of TM in national health care delivery, ensuring "that the necessary regulatory and legal mechanisms are created for promoting" and maintaining good practice, that access is equitable, and that the authenticity, safety and efficacy of therapies are assured. A national TM policy is urgently needed in those developing countries where the population depends largely on TM for health care, but without its having been well-evaluated or integrated into the national health system. Many developed countries, are now considering such policy in taking CAM issues. Presently, with the, exception of China, the Democratic People's Republic of Korea, the Republic of Korea and Vietnam, full integration has not taken place. In many countries, national assessment will therefore be needed to ascertain which TM/CAM modalities can best be integrated into the national health care system.

Health Care Delivery in Nigeria

Health care has become a major concern to various governments, and private organisations due to its importance to human existence. This is the reason why a huge amount of money is being spent worldwide to provide good health care services. However, the quality of these services varies from one place to another and from one country to another. It is adequate in developed countries like Britain, USA, Germany and France while poor in developing countries like Nigeria, Ghana and Liberia. High standard of health care delivery of nation connotes her high standard of living.

Health care delivery *per* se is the delivery of health care services provided by the various health care centres to patients in need of them. In Nigeria, health care delivery is inadequate and needs a serious attention. Efforts made by the government to address this problem are simply not satisfactory. In 1993, there were 5,208 people per doctor while in 2003, the country-had an infant mortality rate of 71 deaths per 1,000 live births. Around 2.7 per cent of the country's GDP was spent on health care in 1989. Health services are accessible to wealthier urban dwellers only. Malaria, yaws, and yellow fever are prevalent or rife.

Health care services in Nigeria are delivered through the primary, secondary and tertiary care centres. The primary health centre is the first port of call when seeking for medical attention. The objective of this primary health centre is to bring medical services close to the doorstep of rural dwellers. Village health workers and birth attendants render such services. Examples of primary health centre include maternity homes, health centers, *et cetera*. Medical cases beyond their powers are referred to secondary health centres.

On the other hand, secondary health care centres include private and general hospitals. They manage cases referred to them from primary health centres. The urban centralisation of these centres enables them to serve the major cities. Cases that cannot be treated in these hospitals are referred to tertiary health centres. Tertiary health care centres are specialist or referral centres where medical cases that cannot be handled at secondary health care centres are referred. Examples include teaching hospitals and specialist hospitals.

The health care centres in the country spread over rural and urban settlements across the nation, with majority of these centres located in urban settlements. Health care delivery systems at these centres are poor, inadequate and not keeping with modern medical services in the developed world.

Over time, joint efforts have been made by the federal government and state as a pivot to improve health care delivery system throughout the country. Some of these efforts include the current launching of national health insurance scheme (NHIS), roll back malaria programmes, polio eradication programmes, building of new medical centres, procurement of vaccines, and purchase of modern medical equipment, among others.

Problems Affecting Health Care Delivery

Despite these efforts, health care delivery service in Nigeria is still far from being satisfactory. Problems affecting health care delivery in the country include:

1. *Inadequate Medical Personnel*

There is dearth of inadequate medical personnel in health institutions. The doctors and the supporting medical personnel are so few for the country's population. This problem affects the larger population who dwell more in rural areas than urban cities. This is because the few available medical personnel tend to live in the cities in preference to rural areas.

2.   *Unequal Distribution of Medical Facilities*

Most of our health institutions are located in the cities with few or none sited in some rural areas. This poses a major problem to the larger population, which live in the rural areas.

3.   *Lack of Adequate Access Roads*

Furthermore, lack of access roads interconnecting the communities in rural areas to the cities is a serious problem. Most of these roads are in deplorable state. This makes it difficult for rural dwellers to get access to the nearest available modern health care especially in emergency situations.

4.   *Poverty*

Poverty is a major problem facing most rural dwellers. Even when the patient finally managed to get to the hospitals located in the city, the rural dwellers cannot afford the cost of treatment and drugs. This makes some patients to be discouraged from seeking medical care and subsequently resort to traditional means which are considered cheaper. More often than not, the services of these traditional doctors are inadequate. When their services fail, patient will be left with no other option than to find their way to the hospital at a time that might be too late to be assisted.

5.   *Ignorance and Cultural Barriers*

Ignorance, superstition and religious beliefs constitute a problem to health care delivery. Patients in this category do not believe in modern concept of diseases and health care services for instance, some parents deny their children immunisation against killer diseases. Reason for this is attributed to their belief that vaccines meant for immunisation also contain family planning drugs.

In summary, health is considered to be a reflection of a country's economy. That is why government spends a huge amount of money to improve health care delivery in the country. Despite some of these laudable efforts, the system is still far from being satisfactory. The poor health care delivery system in Nigeria is attributable to inadequate medical personnel, poverty, ignorance, superstition and religious belief, among others.

In order to enhance the quality of health care delivery in the country, the government need to develop rural areas and ensure equitable distribution of medical facilities to various communities, train more medical personnel into available health institutions, construct access roads to link communities with urban areas and organise health campaign to counter ignorance and superstition, among other measures. In addition the training and utilisation of traditional health practitioners in primary health care, working in close collaboration with conventional health staff, can be expected to contribute substantially, to obtaining more practical, effective, and culturally acceptable health systems for the diverse communities in the country.

Endnotes

1.   The striking differences between the developed and the developing world in terms of health care are reflected in the differing life expectancy of their populations and mortality rates.

2.   The term complementary seems to make a less ambitious claim than alternative which appear rather hostile, hence the former is more preferred, while the terms unofficial, fringe and folk are derogatory.

3.   The highest ethical standards were imposed on the physicians, who took the celebrated oath usually attributed to Hippocrates and which is still in use today (see the full text and the modernised version of the oath in the Appendix).

4.   What we conventionally name as Islamic or Arabic medicine is not a genuine medical system indigenous to the Arabian Peninsula. Islamic medicine was not developed solely by Arabs, since Christians, Jews, and, mainly, Muslims of diverse ethnical origins contributed to its development. Nevertheless, whatever their religious confession and geographical location, these scholars and physicians all worked in the sphere of Islamic hegemony and employed the Arabic language as a vehicle for their literary works.

The history of Western medicine cannot be fully understood without medieval Islamic medicine, since medieval Islamic culture was the source of European philosophic and scientific ideas during the period between the decline of the Classical period and the beginning of the Renaissance, formerly known as the "Dark Ages" . Medieval Islamic medicine continues to exist even today as a formal medical practice in some Asian countries such as India and Pakistan, under the name *Unani* (Greek, "medicine"), alongside modern Western medicine and the *Ayurvedic* tradition.

5.   See Appendix on PHC.

Traditional Medicine and Classes of Traditional Healers

From too much zeal for what is new and contempt for what is old, from putting knowledge before wisdom, science before art; cleverness before common sense; Good Lord deliver us – Sir Robert Hutchinson, 1871-1960

Traditional medicine, like orthodox medicine, aims at healing or preventing diseases. In this respect, both types of medicine have the same objective, but they differ in their concepts of the causes of disease, their approach to healing as well as in the methods of treatment used. Traditional medicine places greater emphasis on the spiritual and supernatural causes of disease and forces of healing than orthodox medicine. As a result, the traditional healers are consulted not only in terms of sickness but also when an evil omen is suspected or when misfortune such as accidents, deaths, losses, etc, occur or are to be averted. These practices may also be employed to secure fame or success in life adventures. In general, traditional medicine is deeply rooted in the culture of the people that use it, and as a result, it is closely linked to their beliefs.

Traditional medicine comprises several unconventional approaches to healing and health, many of which are now thought to complement conventional medicine. Some of these medicaments or practices have gained widespread acceptance and approval by both conventional doctors and the general public, but many others are still viewed with suspicion and occasionally outright hostility by the established medical profession.

There is no denying the fact that traditional medicine is an integral part of health care delivery in Nigeria. About 80% of Nigerian homes, at one time or the other, employ the services of a traditional medical practitioner [TMP]. According to the National Investigative Committee on Traditional and Alternative Medicine (NICTAM) Report of 1985, there were 200,000 traditional healers in the country at the time. The number has certainly increased in the last 17 years. It is also true that traditional medicine not only influences the society deeply and brings recovery of health to millions of people at low cost but also creates havoc for millions of others at high cost. While it can boast truthfully about many herbs with curative potencies and great pharmacological value, it is also a tool for deception and various forms of immorality and social catastrophes such as murder, enmity, abortion, psychological and psychiatric disorder, profiteering and abuse by charlatans.

Because both the government and the good traditional medical practitioners have not been able to insulate the profession, from corruption, abuse and invasion by unscrupulous elements, all kinds of people such as the unemployed, the criminal, the psychologically unbalanced and the physically handicapped hide under the pretext of traditional medicine and use it to dupe desperate victims. Presently, several groups of traditional healers exist in the country. They are widespread in every hamlet, village, town or city such that they cannot be easily censored. A few of them run stationary practices of varying size waiting for people to come for consultation, while the majority travel from place to place seeking patients in marketplaces, motor parks, religious centres or in their homes for medical services. Some of them act as general practitioners able to prescribe for a number of different ailments, while others are specialists for one type of disease or the other. In general, they include the following classes:

The Spiritualists

These are practitioners of spirit possession cult with its origin from the pagan times. They claim to communicate with the spirits and to intervene on behalf of the patients for the treatment of miscarriages, infertility, personal protection against evil spirits, evil eye, necromancy, witchcraft, etc.

The Magicians

They are traditional healers highly skilled in the art of magic and deception, and they usually administer drugs which are mainly of herbal or animal ingredients. They prepare love potions and give medicines for immunisation or prophylaxis against snake bites or scorpion sting, among others.

Barber-Surgeons

The barber-surgeons are specialists involved in performing cupping (bloodletting), lancing of abscesses, swellings or cauterisation, uvulectomy, circumcision and scarification or tribal marks. Cupping (bloodletting) involves making of deep incision on the affected part of the body, usually where a swelling has occurred. The impure or 'bad' blood is then sucked out with the aid of a horn (or cup) open at both ends. Modern medicine discourages the surgical activity of the barber-surgeons because of predisposition to infection, haemorrhage and debility resulting from unhygienic practices and ignorance of body anatomy (structure). The barber-surgeons are also notoriously known among orthodox medical practitioners for their popular *'gishiri* cut'. This procedure involves an incision (surgical cut) on the anterior and (rarely) posterior aspect of the vagina as a treatment for a variety of conditions, including dyspareunia (painful sexual intercourse), small introitus (vaginal opening), vaginismus, infertility (childlessness), amenorrhoae, (absence of menses), prolonged obstructed labour and intersex disorders, etc. The cut usually result in haermorrhage (bleeding), and if deep, result in fistula (abnormal opening) between vagina and rectum (recto-vaginal fistula-RVF) or between vagina and urinary bladder (vesico-vaginal fistula-VVF).

Traditional Birth Attendants

A Traditional birth attendant (TBA) or traditional midwife is usually an elderly woman, who administers antenatal care, conducts deliveries and also looks after the mother and the child in the post-natal period (i.e. after delivery). She gives advice on diet, may prescribe herbs (topical, oral, powdery or smoky). She may also pass restrictions to the lactating mother, such as to throwaway colostrums (early breast milk), to remain indoors, take daily hot baths, sleep on heated beds, and eat food rich in pepper and potassium or sodium salts so as to protect the mother from cold and aid her return to normalcy, especially in the reproductive parts. These procedures are potentially dangerous. Unhygienic cutting off of umbilicus is a common cause of neonatal tetanus infection and death. The hot baths cause severe superficial burns and may lead to dehydration.

It has also been pointed by Professor E.H.O. Parry in his book, *Principles of Medicine in Africa,* that, Northern Nigerian has one of the highest incidence of post partum cardiac failure in the world. This is due to the volume load from eating the customary sodium-rich pap *(kunun kanwa),* and the cardiovascular demands of heat, both climatic and traditionally self-imposed. The condem-nation of colostrums (early breast milk) by the traditional birth attendant is condemnable, because it is scientifically found to be richer in nutrients and antibodies (which fight against infection) than breast milk that is produce afterwards. However, the training and integration of traditional birth attendants (TBA) is being successfully attempted in many parts of the country so that they can improve their techniques using modern hygienic methods and guidelines.

Herbalists

These are specialists in administration of herbal medicines for curative and preventive purposes. Sometimes, they also use animal ingredients. The herbalists are the main streamline of traditional medical practitioners, and sometimes their name seems to encompass all other traditional healers. Presently, they are the initiators and leaders of the movement for recognition of traditional practitioners as legitimate medical practitioners. This form of complementary medicine has been practised through the centuries, and probably from several thousands of years ago. Depending on the plant and the treatment, the whole plant or individual parts can be used in the remedy.

Generally, practitioners used seeds, fruit flowers, leaves, stems, and barks of plants and herbs in preparing remedies. The commonest form of remedy is the infusion, the fresh herb or plant boiled and the water strained and sipped like tea. The tincture (one part of the herb or plant mixed with five parts of alcohol) is also a common form of therapy. Herbal practitioners also prescribe use of herbs; in suppository, inhalant, lotion, tablet, and liquid forms. Many diseases can be treated with herbal medicines. Some commonly treated conditions include colds and influenza, insomnia, and nausea and vomiting. Certainly their claims have been duly substantiated as numerous scientific laboratories throughout the world have and are continuing to analyse and evaluate the herbs advocated by the herbalists. Many of the herbs are found to be active and of therapeutic value, and called for adoption, but there also many areas of lapses and excesses, which called for rejection.

Bonesetters

The bonesetters are specialists in the treatment of bone fractures, dislocations and sprains. They treat fractures by tying pieces of wood or straight stems (as splints) with a fibrous plant or rope round the broken bone on the body surface and applying traditional medicaments to the area. Sometimes, the bonesetters fracture the leg of a chicken at the same time as treating a human fracture, the chicken being given the same treatment as the patient. It is believed that when the chicken is able to walk again, the patient's fracture will have healed sufficiently for him to try walking with the bad leg. In certain occasions, when the procedure proved unsuccessful, the bonesetters may re-fracture the affected bone and reset it again.

This can be repeated until the bonesetter is satisfied with the fracture healing.

Traditional bonesetters are highly respected and their services are often preferred to modern orthopaedic surgeons, because some people feel that their limbs could be amputated (removed) if they go to hospital for treatment of fracture. It is most commonly known that the traditional bonesetters often mismanage fractures of their patients and such patients (usually brought lately to the hospital after the fracture has become complicated) may ultimately require either amputation to prevent spread of gangrene or further surgery to correct allied deformities.

In modern medical practice, once there is fracture, attention is also given to other associated and indeed delicate structures such as veins and arteries, which carries blood to and from the area and the nerve fibres, which transmit impulses to and from the area. Neglecting these structures and paying attention to the bone only, as traditional bonesetters often do, can and usually lead to death of the limb and spread of infection to the whole body, which may result in either amputation of the limb or death of the person concerned.

In the case of compound or open fractures (in which the bone protrudes through the skin), it must be emphasised that such patient should be referred to orthodox surgeons who not only attempts to knit together the broken edges or pieces of a bone, but also gives serious consideration to restoration of the function of the bone after healing, prevention of infection, severe loss of blood or serious threats to life. It has been observed in many occasions that some bonesetter's treatment of complicated fractures has resulted in permanent deformation, which would have been prevented, had the patient been referred to a hospital.

However, traditional bonesetters are useful in health care provided they accept to recognise their limitations in handling certain fractures. Some traditional bonessetters appear competent in the management of simple uncomplicated fractures. If they can utilise the benefits of modern medicine through such investigative techniques like x-rays (to be taken before and after setting the bone), they will undoubtedly' improve their performance. Evaluation and training of such healers could prove to be useful area for integration.

The Religious Healers

A religious healer acting as a traditional medical practitioner is highly respected and is one of the most frequently consulted and most trusted of the healers. He bases his authority and power on the religious texts and the spiritual power of his prayers. He gives washed scriptural writings on wooden slates and verses wrapped in animal skin leather as amulet or charm as medication, either for preventive or curative purposes. The hallmark of his treatment is prayers, incantations or supplication to the Almighty God as the source of cure and healing.

Until recently, the position of the religious healer in the traditional society was unchallenged. But due to their excesses, being a haven of consultation by persons engaged in robbery, dupery, professional fraud (coded '419'), armed robbery, prostitution - *the very evils which true religion condemns and rejects,* they are losing their grip among the youths and the elite in the society. Some times ago, relevant government agencies has clamped down on many religious healers because of their' exaggerated claim to possessing miraculous healing prowess through all forms of advert in both electronic and print media. However, some of the genuine preachers as a result of their dramatic performance in exorcism (driving out evil spirits from possessed persons by prayers and the use of authentic medicaments such as honey, dates, nigella seed *(habbatus-sawdat),* etc, are bringing prestige to the religious healer and restoring his traditional status. Modern medicine, though silent on these matters relating to evil spirits or *jinn,* provides an alternative in the growing field of psychology, psychoanalysis and psychiatry.

Diviners

The diviners are group of traditional healers who specialise in the art of prophesy (that is, foretelling about future events), analysis of dreams, incantations and sacrifices in the diagnosis and treatment of their patients. Some of them use handful of seeds or cowries, which are thrown on the ground to form a pattern from which they derive their mystical knowledge and prowess. This form of practice cannot be assessed scientifically as such ethno-medical research does not extend to this aspect of traditional medicine.

However, it is observed that some diviners play on the intelligence of their patients by making a careful study of their condition and disposition to arrive at their diagnosis and method of treatment. For example, a troubled woman coming to the diviner (by way of psychological deduction) is likely to have matrimonial problems in the same way a businessman may have problems with his business. But despite the subjectivity of this form of approach or deduction, their patients are usually satisfied, perhaps because in most cases the consultation was for a psychological ailment which is simply cured by counseling, psychotherapy, and reassurance.

Traditional Drugs and Methods of Treatment

The use of plants as remedies is common and widespread in Nigeria. Plant parts being used include the bark, leaves, roots, flowers, fruits and seeds. They are either used as fresh or dried in the form of decoctions or concoction (mixture) - when more than one plant species are used for the preparation of the drug thereby enhancing the claim of *'remedy for all maladies'*. Herbs commonly used by TMPs include *dogonyaro, sanga-sanga, magarya, soborodo, kalgo* and *sabara* among Hausas; *orin ata, gbogboleshe, agunmu jedi-jedi, ira* and *agunmuiba;* among Yorubas; *gongorise, ube* and *nchaun* among Igbos; *gilwade* and *caski,* among Fulanis; *kangalgaski, lubasar* and *kulu'u* among Kanuris, etc. It is noteworthy that each tribe and community has their own varieties of drugs. Therefore, traditional drugs vary from one community to another and that explains its unconventional status.

Traditional drugs are used in the treatment of abdominal pain, dysentery, headache, fever, difficult or prolonged labour, body pains and improvement of sexual performance, while some of the herbs in combination with other herbs are used in making concoction *(tsime)* for the treatment of many diseases.

Various routes of drug administration are employed; oral, topical, anal, vaginal, nasal fumigation and smoking. Use of animal ingredients is also common among the various classes of traditional healers.

Animal parts being used include horn, hoof, claws, hair, peak, fats, bone, teeth, flesh, tail, skin, etc. Sometimes even visibly, nonexistent parts of an animal are claimed to be used in preparing medicines. Such things may include *legs of a worm, the bones of fly, the penis of a snake, fatty tissue of a female mosquito, breast of a chameleon,* etc. At times, the healer will claim to have used or direct the patient to provide, as part of the ingredients for preparing a potion, hardly accessible materials such as the teeth of a virgin leopard, saliva of a young bat, sperm of a fertile lion, egg of a crocodile, etc.

The traditional practitioners also use other means of diagnosis and treatment. These include physical means, such as history taking, examination, analysis of urine, faeces or saliva (by using their sensory organs for the observation of colour, smell, etc) and non-physical methods such as divination, spirit possession, exorcism, sacrifices, use of astrological signs, and analysis of dreams. These methods, though unacceptable to modern medicine, their effects on the individual, both physical and psychological, cannot be denied.

Acceptable methods of treatment used by' the traditional healers include exercise, massage (somatotherapy), relaxation therapy, aromatherapy, visualisation, meditation, psychotherapy, counseling, environmental manipulation, nutritional and occupational therapy and rehabilitation.

Criticisms against Traditional Medical Practice

What has been said heretofore demonstrates that traditional medicine comprises a mass of practices ranging from the worthless and harmful to highly effective remedies. Far from being a deliberate wish to cast aspersions on traditional medicine, which, as emphasised earlier, constitute the foundation from which the so-called modern medicine evolved, this is a fair and bold attempt to point out the ill-effects of this system or the other for the sake of research and objectivity, and overall human progress.

In essence, this should not be seen as mere criticism but stimulation. The integration of modern system with traditional system of medicine must be achieved by the coordinating effects of a modern scientist to study, and with open mind, the rudiments of traditional medicine and *vice versa*. In the end, this will help in fact-finding, by sorting out those that deserves confirmation or condemnation within the spectrum of any of the systems.

Nevertheless, some of the criticisms directed against the practice of traditional medicine in Nigeria can be summarised as follows:

Poor Concept of Disease

In traditional medicine, disease is considered a visitation of evil and malevolent spirits or punishment of the Almighty God for sins of omission or commission. Consequently, appropriate measures are not put in place to address emergency and physically existing or verifiable situations.

Association of Treatment with Unhealthy Practices

Association of treatment with cultic practices, invocation of spirits, rituals, incantations and sacrifices (which may even involve human life) and other mystic practices, tend to wreak havoc on the society leading to a chain of negative events which affect mental, social, and physical health of the individual.

Lack of Precision on Drug Dosage and Duration of Treatment

In traditional medical practice, there is no conventional drug package for treatment of disease. Consequently, there is tendency for overdose or underdose of the drugs leading to disastrous consequences. In contrast to traditional medicine, orthodox practice provides specific periods for drug use and measuring duration of treatment whether palliative, conservative, elective or emergency.

Unpreparedness to Control Side Effects

Traditional medical practitioners have sent many patients to their graves by giving those drugs whose side effects they could not control. Example is the case of a patient who procured diarrhoea-inducing drug without a provision to stop the diarrhoea. Consequently, the person became dehydrated and died as a result of uncontrolled diarrhoea. The same problem applies in the use of traditional herbs as aphrodisiacs (substances meant to improve sexual performance or potency like prolongation of penile erection) which may eventually lead to impotence. In contrast, modern practice provides a standby alternative to combat toxicity or side effects in the use of drugs. For instance, chlorpheniramine (piriton), an anti-histamine, is used to counteract the excessive itching effect produced by chloroquine in the treatment of malaria.

Unhygienic Practices

In contrast to modern practice, the materials used, the preparation, procedures and places of operation in traditional practice are usually unhygienic. This paves way for unmitigated disaster and calamity. Drug packages (wrapped in dirty materials), without preservative and consumer information may, with time become real and lethal poisons.

Poor Storage Facilities

Usually after preparation of traditional drugs, they are stored in earthen ware pots, tortoise shell, gourds, horse hooves, horns, bamboos stem, calabashes, etc. Whatever attribute "tradition confer on these types of containers, they are not good storage facilities and therefore, cannot provide full protection to the drugs against external or internal hazards. Such hazards include mixture with organic or inorganic chemicals, effects of temperature, sunlight, micro-organisms, dust particles, etc. The effect of any of these could lead to spoilage of the medicaments and consequently, therapeutic failure and or introduction of new disease to the patient.

Ignorance of Biochemical Effects of the Herbs

Administration of any herb which has adverse biochemical effects on the body, unknown to both the healer and the patient, can lead to calamitous effects. For instance, digitalis, quinine, reserpine and atropine are modified traditional drugs whose adverse side effects can lead to excessive activity of the heart (arrhythmias), cardiac arrest and sudden death. This cannot be the case in modern practice, where an up-to-date knowledge of drug is obtained and clinical trials conducted several times before marketing and use.

Itinerancy

In contrast to orthodox practitioners, most traditional medicine practitioners are itinerant healers who travel from one place to another looking for patients. Professor Badoe and his colleagues in page 2 of their book, *The Principles and Practice of Surgery in the Tropics,* described such healers as

> ignorant, unscrupulous and often brutal men who wandered from place to place and fled before their failure and mishaps could catch up with them.

Since traditional healers do not run a permanent station or clinic, there is no way their patients can establish correspondence with them in a feedback system. Thus, they lack commitment to patients, acceptance of responsibility for their actions and respect for the rule of law, which are all observable in their modern counterparts.

Lack of Code of Conduct and Ethics

In traditional medicine, some healers procure abortion, engage in witchcrafts, poisoning, psychic manipulation and profiteering with little or no control as long as they likes, because they are not ethic-oriented or regulated by a diligent professional body. Sometimes, even normal healthy patients visit them to seek the negative benefits of their medicine (what is called 'black magic') against their perceived, imaginary or real enemies! In orthodox practice, every practitioner must undertake the pledge to "maintain the utmost respect for human life from its beginning, even under threat, and he will not use his medical knowledge contrary to the laws of humanity". Therefore, orthodox medicine is regulated by a well-defined universal code of conduct that guides the practice of the profession in all parts of the world.

Secrecy in Medical Training and Practice

In traditional medicine, the whole thing is shrouded in mystery. Training is either by guarded apprenticeship or by family inheritance. As a result of this guarding of information (secrecy), truth and error are equally transmitted without probity or criticism. In comparison, training in the orthodox practice is well-publicised, organised and official. Every physician is recognised based on his/her qualification. Knowledge is transmitted easily, handled with discretion, and updated with the advancement attained by research and scholarship.

Lack of Division of Labour, Specialisation and Diversification

There is lack of adequate or organised division of labour in the traditional setting. The healer is the *alpha* and *omega*. Consequently, traditional medicine moves slowly and reluctantly towards development and still retains some elements of primitivity. This is in contrast with the rapidly advancing fields of orthodox medicine (in view of the remarkable achievements recorded in space medicine, genetic engineering, neuro-surgery, and other sub-specialties, etc). In modern medical practice, health care coverage is a product of various professionals: physicians, surgeons, dentists, nurses, midwives, pharmacists, community health workers, psychiatrists, physio-therapists, anaesthetists and scientists, among others. Hence, specialisation, diversification and division of labour are well-developed in orthodox practice.

Prescriptions are Blindly Holistic

In orthodox medical practice, certain drugs are allowed for some patients but contraindicated in some group of people (such as the pregnant mothers, children, diabetes, hypertensive or ulcer patients, etc). Lack of such system of contraindication in traditional practice makes the patients insecure *(anything can happen)*. And when it does, one can imagine the consequences!

Irrational Approach to the Causes of Diseases

Traditional medicine is irrational, that is, does not depend on reason, and is often mythical in explaining the cause of diseases, since knowledge from the handouts of traditional healers reveals that evil spirits, witches; cruel ancestors and so on, are the real causes of diseases and not necessarily typhoid or malaria. This belief also tends to promote the concept of 'my enemy syndrome' which ascribes the cause of disease to one's real or imaginary enemies, thereby a vicious circle of chasing shadows (rather than the real agents of a disease process) took over the search for cure leading to unwanted delays, and the onset of irreversible complication.

Orthodox medicine, on the other hand, *a relatively safe one for that matter,* produces rational and scientific explanations of the causes of diseases based on physical and attested facts or tangible factors such as bacteria, viruses, fungi and parasites, reached through a coordinated system of history taking, clinical examination and series of investigations. It is also cognisant of non-tangible factors (external forces) such as environmental and social factors, life events, genetic predisposition, etc.

False Claim of Remedy for all Maladies

It is a common occurrence to see a TMP giving undue and exaggerated advert to his skills, medical prowess or drugs, claiming that a particular concoction possesses remedy for all maladies - *abdominal pain, headache, diarrhoea, ear ache, conjunctivitis, backache, hypertension, liver disease,* etc. There will be no end to such unregulated, unguided and unguarded propaganda and ruse, which to borrow the words of James Hadley Chase, "If you believe this, you'll believe anything"! Seriously speaking, this is one of the greatest setbacks of traditional practice as many practitioners claim ability and expertise in handling all conditions of ill health under heaven. Sometimes, they ascribe curative power on a single drug over several unrelated and nonexisting disorders.

Conscientiously and consciously, no one should claim ability or expertise to cure all or any type of disease. What is even more worrisome is the manner some healers go about it, particularly in relation to media adverts, by arrogantly parading themselves as 'healers'. Some of them unequivocally claim to provide guarantee of recovery within a specific period for anyone who goes to them. This is absurd and ridiculous because the power of healing is divine. In other words, only God can guarantee recovery from illness. In orthodox practice, it is deemed unethical for any practitioner to engage in self-advertisement either directly or indirectly, and breach of the code is liable to disciplinary actions by the appropriate organs or authorities. Thus, a genuine medical practitioner can only guarantee the best of his/her skills and services *(as Hippocrates' declared, "according to my ability and judgement")* but cannot negotiate on the basis of providing absolute cure. In actual sense, cure depends on certain natural factors outside the total control of the physician.

Lack of Meritocracy

Merits elude traditional medicine because its intellectual basis is not institutionalised, so no accredited degree or qualification. Training is through unspecified period of apprenticeship and "order of merit" correlates with increasing age. Usually, expertise is attained at old age. The profession is practised in close knitted communities where the traditional healer stays, and as such it is believed that their integrity and competence were most likely controlled to some extent by the social relationships of their place of residence. The usage of the title 'doctor' (abbreviated Dr) for themselves is seen by many orthodox practitioners as illegal, self-acclaimed and usurpation of a title they do not deserve, since they do not pass through any rigorous training or formal schooling.

Misdiagnosis and Mismanagement

It is common to find a traditional healer making a diagnosis of 'stomach trouble' (whatever that means) and managing his patient along that line. In the actual sense, 'stomach trouble' could mean indigestion, a peptic ulcer, or cancer of the stomach or intestinal obstruction or typhoid perforation, liver disease or any other thing. The misdiagnosis is due to the fact that the body anatomy and pathology of certain diseases is not known to the overzealous traditional medical practitioner. As a result, therefore, he tends to treat the symptom rather than the actual disease. This situation sometimes leads to a lot of problems and further complications.

Other Problems

These include irrational use of many herbs (multi-component mixture or poly-pharmacy), lack of insight into the other consequences of drug administration (such as drug-drug interactions), hostility among healers, lack of referral systems, lack of health education, physical assaults on patients, ignorance of body anatomy (structure) and function (physiology), lack of conventional treatment modality, exploitation of patients (through fraudulent means, dishonesty and deception), absence of scientific thinking, paranoia and uncritical acceptance of cause of disease ('my enemy syndrome'), lack of understanding of how therapeutic effects may be measured ('all or none mentally'), among others.

Why Do People Patronise Traditional Healers?

In view of the many problems associated with some aspects of traditional medical practice in Nigeria, one may begin to ask why the traditional healers are getting more patronage even from educated elite in the society. The factors are not far-fetched, and include the following:

The Socio-Cultural Barrier

Although there is the recognition that health is a fundamental human right, there is denial of this right to millions of people who are caught in the vicious circle of poverty, ignorance and disease. A very high proportion of the population particularly in rural areas does not have ready access to health services, which seems to favour only the privileged few and educated urban dwellers. In addition, there are in existence social and political structures, which are biased in favour of urban settlements. These include availability of electricity, accessible roads, potable water, improved sanitation, manpower (for example, preference of urban to rural settlement by doctors), etc.

Again, certain elements within the organisational framework of modern health services are at variance with the cultural beliefs, values and behavioural patterns of the local people. Even among African elites, diseases are always related to one's enemies and adversaries and the need to appease God or gods by prayers and rituals respectively or use of charms and amulets plays an important role. In fact, situations abound where some elites consult traditional healers in secret but boast of using orthodox medicine in the open.

Another important and potent barrier-factor is language. English which is the common medium of communication for orthodox practitioners and the *lingua franca* is only known by a relatively small percentage of the population. The use of interpreter may appeal to the orthodox practitioner but most patients resent such means of communication because they feel that their medical problems cannot be appreciated by the doctor through a *second-hand* informant. Since these socio-cultural distances do not exist between traditional healers and their clients as to hamper effective utilisation of health services, people preferred going to traditional healing homes.

Sophistication of Orthodox Medical Services

Orthodox medicine is highly sophisticated and bureaucratised. The graded steps in management; history-taking, clinical examinations, treatment, referral, clinic follow-ups, co-management with other specialists, etc, are considered by many to be 'too cumbersome' in contrast to the 'simple' approach of traditional medicine. This creates additional delays in seeking prompt medical services. The patient may have travelled long distances to the hospital and could have waited for several hours before being seen in an environment which for many rural dwellers is strange, with relatively sophisticated people and their machines all about to focus their attention on him. All these things, which are not strange to the medical practitioner, may be frightening to the patient. As a result, local people referred to tertiary health centers resent being teleguided, rebuked or humbled when they meet a highly institutionalised service. This discourages them from going to hospitals and diverts them to traditional healing homes.

Accessibility

Traditional medical practitioners bring health services to the doorsteps of the people. Despite the current national policy on health which has at its cornerstone, primary health care based on the Alma-Ata Declaration, modern services are not as close or accessible to the local people as the traditional medicine. For instance, the fact that Nigeria has a proportion of nomads[1] in their population creates logistics problems in making health services accessible to all. Because of their constant movement and dispersion, it is difficult for conventional health services to be made available to them. But this is not a problem for traditional medical care because they either have their own traditional healers among them or come across them through the communities they pass through.

Affordability

Traditional healers provide comparatively cheaper services which local people can afford. They collect as their fee material gifts (goats, palm oil, millet, chicken, yam, etc) which the local people can always afford. Sometimes, the healers often offer credit services or totally prefer spiritual to material reward. In contrast to traditional medicine, modern health care services are costly.

The cost is high as a result of modern health technology which in many cases, is inappropriate and irrelevant to the immediate needs of the rural people in developing countries[2]. Recently, the cost of modern health care services has increased due to the demand for improved health workers' welfare and higher cost of basic commodities, fuel and agricultural products.

Lack of Education and Awareness

Many people, though they have some form of education, may be genuinely ignorant about health matters. For instance, people do not appreciate the dangers of drug overdose, poor hygiene associated with traditional drugs, the placebo (psychological) effect produced by many herbs, etc. And the fact remains unknown to many people that for many diseases, there may be spontaneous recovery with time. Such people therefore ascribe natural healing to some traditional herbs even when such effects are unrelated! Many patients also seek for traditional treatment because they are unable to determine whether this form of medication or procedure is harmful, beneficial or useless. Others seek traditional medical health care services because of the community belief that certain types of diseases such as mental illnesses, convulsions, epilepsy, etc cannot be treated by orthodox doctors and can only respond to traditional cures.

Misconceptions About Modern Medicine

Many local people misconstrue the good aims of modern medicine for example, in the management of bone fractures, there is growing resentment against orthopaedic-surgeons whom are said to favour amputation to any other method of management. There is also a cry of despair in consulting psychiatrists based on the notion that 'there is no cure for mental illness in modern medicine, since orthodox doctors do not believe *injinn* or witchcraft.

Prejudice against Modern Medicine

Since modern medicine is termed 'Western', everything associated with it is viewed with contempt and distrust by many local people. For example, family planning and immunisation services in many parts of Northern Nigeria are considered as Western plots against the local people for racial, political or religious ill motives. Consequently, many people prefer traditional healers to orthodox practitioners.

Exaggerated Show of Confidence

Many traditional practitioners sometimes boast of feats that are almost impossible in an effort to reassure their patients, improve their morale or boost their own reputation. Sometimes, they make practical demonstration of their power. For example, Professor Abayomi Sofowora recounted an experience he witnessed in which a traditional healer revived a moribund chicken by striking it with an amulet as a demonstration of his ability to revive a dying human being! In turn, the patients' belief in them and their mystical prowess increased and remain unshaken. In contrast, the orthodox doctor guided by his code of ethics and ethos cannot engage in self-advertisement or alluring demonstration of his expertise. He relies on his experimentally proven medicament, his skills or expert ability in diagnosis and the use of readily available diagnostic tests. Sometimes, he may refer his patients to specialists or co-manage them with other physicians. This 'complacency' and humility can lead to doubts in the patient's mind as to the doctor's ability in handling his medical problems and he may eventually decide to patronise the traditional healer.

Attention   to   Patients   and   Good Psychotherapy

Many traditional healers are good psychotherapists. They have ample time for their patients, are ready to listen, and discuss extensively with them. They speak to their patients politely and using a local language which they understand best. This gives the patients a feeling of reassurance, self-esteem, respect and comfortability. In contrast, the orthodox doctor or pharmacist may not have ample time for a particular patient in most cases. The heavy load of patients waiting in a long queue for consultation at the clinic denies him the opportunity of a long talk with or excellent psychotherapy for his patients. In fact, there are some health workers who may not even give their patients the adequate attention necessary for history-taking, instead they rush to prescribe drugs for them while the patient is midway explaining his problems! This situation seems to discourage many patients from visiting the hospital.

Holistic Concept of Health

One of the fundamental errors of modern medicine is its mechanistic concept of life. This is to say, living organisms are regarded as living machines consisting of separate parts. It believes that all aspects of living organisms can be understood by reducing them to their smaller constituents, and by studying the mechanisms through which these operate or interact. As a result of this view, orthodox doctors seem to ignore the emotional or spiritual aspects of health and healing and concentrate more on the physical.

On the other hand, the holistic approach treats the person as entire unit rather than as separate individual parts. In this, it attempts to bring emotional, social, physical and spiritual dimensions of the person's being into harmony and emphasises the role of therapy or treatment which stimulates the persons' own healing process. This approach, which seems to highlight the interaction between the living body and the spirit, seems to offer to the patients of traditional healers a sort of direction, and a sense of inner peace and happiness that favours improved immunity and recuperative healing process[3].

Endnotes

1. Nomads are members of a tribe or people that move from place to place and have no permanent homes. The Fulanis constitute the commonest nomadic group among other tribes in Nigeria.

2. However, efforts are being made by the Government to place emphasis on Primary Health Care which requires little technology.

3. However, on the face of mounting evidence, orthodox medicine has accepted the role of the diverse factors on health. It is only recently that WHO admitted to this deficiency and makes the confession;

    "The limitation of a mechanistic view of health are now becoming apparent and this has been reinforced by a new awareness of ecology". See "The Relevance of the Concept of Spiritual Health" in *The Medicare Medical Journal,* Vol. 5, No. 10, pp. 11.

Modern Medicine and the Orthodox Medical Practitioner

Undoubtedly, modern medicinie has made and is still making tremendous and ccommendable progress Undeniably too, it represents the later stage in the developmental milestone or evolutionary stage of traditional medicine. In essence, modern medicine is neither Western nor Eastern but a culmination of man's quest for health through the ages, gleaning from the diverse cultures of many peoples, and later from biological and natural sciences, and more recently from social, behavioural and genetic sciences.

From ancient Chinese medicine, regarded as the earliest to Indian *(Ayuverdic)*, Egyptian up to the Greek and Arab *(Unani-Tibb)* medicine, one can appreciate the stages of evolution and development of medicine which gives an overview of man's concern for health and his age-long combat against diseases and afflictions.

A major landmark in the history of modern medicine was however recorded in the 5th century pre-Christian era. This was as a result of the efforts of Greek physicians. The most notably among them was Hippocrates (460-377 BC), traditionally described as the father of modern medicine in recognition of his contribution to the scientific foundation of medicine. It was he, who separated medicine from religio-traditional practice and gave it the form it holds today. He laid down certain principles on which modern medicine is built.

These are:

- That there is no authority except facts;

- That facts should be obtained by accurate observations; and

- That deductions are to be made only from observed facts.

Further development of rational medicine by Greek physicians after Hippocrates greatly improved medical knowledge of the world in the early Christian era. Thereafter, the cultural centre moved to Byzantine empire and then to Arabia.

The underlying Islamic worldview at the time (8th-13th century) gave a fresh vigor and zeal to the development of medical knowledge. Consequently, it was observed that

> the Arabs developed a solid methodology, not only of deriving knowledge through experimentation and reasoning but also for dealing with knowledge that had already been developed by preceding civilisations.

What was called 'medieval' medicine was therefore born, and universities began to function and teach medicine. It was called 'medieval' because at the time in the West, medicine was far from being developed.

In fact, medicine suffered stagnation for a while as new discoveries were frowned upon.

This era of hostility against research and scientific knowledge continued until the beginning of 19th century when scientists revolted against the authority of the church, which at the time was seen to be enslaving intelligence and free development of ideas.

With further advances in scientific knowledge, experimental medicine developed from the tools provided by physiology, pharmacology, biochemistry and other medical sciences. Out of all these, modern medicine grew from the legacy of experiment and experience of not only Western people, but also that of the entire humanity. However, the West must be credited for its rapid development, its intellectual reappraisal and representation to the world in the language of science and modernism.

It would now be said of modern medical practice that its supremacy over the traditional practice is an incontestable reality. Its superiority lies in utilisation of modern science as a tool in the diagnosis, treatment and prevention of diseases and medical disorders.

Another area where modern medicine has an upper hand over the traditional practice borders on the issue of ethics and regulation of professional conduct for practitioners. The Oath of Hippocrates, which is widely believed he imposed on his pupils, remains up till today the code of conduct guiding orthodox practice. It is this Hippocratic school of ethics that has provided a framework for ethical decision-making in medicine for almost 2,500 years.

Every member of the profession endeavour to abide

by the dictates of the Physician's Oath (the modern version of the Hippocratic Oath), which is the foundation of the code of ethics of the profession. Embodied in this oath are the guidelines for behavioural interaction between the practitioner and his clients, colleagues, teachers and the public. Fundamental to these ethical guidelines is the allegiance, which every practitioner owes to the corporate body of the profession.[1]

The corporate body of the medical profession has, by tradition or convention through the ages, assumed the responsibility for maintaining and constantly enhancing the standard of service provided to the public, as well as protecting the profession from unwarranted encroachment by charlatans and quacks. In this way, the medical profession has been from time immemorial and universally still remains, the most learned and the noblest among the original three learned professions.[2]

Another developmental aspect of modern medicine is partnership. Successful medical therapy has always depended on a partnership among the various cadres of health professionals (doctors, pharmacists, nurses, laboratory scientists, social workers and or counsellors) and between them and the clients, which are also categorised (in-patients, out-patients, specialist cases, referrals) for convenience and effectiveness in management.

Modern pharmacology, has also added greater prestige to orthodox practice. Drugs are prepared and tested according to the most vigorous criteria of standardisation, for the sake of safety, efficacy as well as economic efficiency.

However, in spite of the spectacular achievements of modern medicine, it still has a lot of unsolved problems before it. First, although the old code of medical ethics described a duty of beneficence and non-maleficence among many moral precepts, it! now seems inadequate to deal with the complex ethical problems arising from new developments in medicine and the delivery of health care. For example, the spread of human immunodeficiency virus (HIV) has triggered widespread! debate about how much risk to the physician is acceptable in caring for the various categories of patients. If the patient; makes the delivery of health care dangerous, is the physician obliged to treat him or has the patient forfeited his rights.[3]

Apart from dealing with the problems of patients who constitute; risks to the physician, orthodox practice also grapples with the issue of practitioners who poses a risk to their patients. These are doctors with infectious disease; including BIV, those impaired by physical illness (for example, Parkinson's disease), drug or substance abuse, fatigue, old age, psychiatric disorders, overzealous researchers, dishonest doctors or practitioners who exploit their patients, and so on. There are other controversial issues in orthodox practice. These include induced abortion, euthanasia (mercy killing), and organ transplantation, in spite of its promising prospects in this millennium.

In general, given that harm caused by medical treatment amounts to a health problem of considerable magnitude and that *"primum non necere"* (first, do no harm) has been a fundamental tenet of medicine since the era of Hippocrates. It is unacceptable that patients be exposed to unnecessary and avoidable risks. In the same vein, the doctors' position must be secured. They must not be exposed to unnecessary risk, be cheated or deprived of their legitimate entitlements. Even though it has been said that the issue of rights and needs in the doctor-client relationship is often one-sided (that is, the balance of power is unequal in favour of the orthodox practitioners), what is reassuring is that the traditional view of doctors as indefatigable, selfless, all-wise; and error-free superbeings is giving (paving) way to a new view, one based on reality rather than perception. But this is not all.

Another problem which modern medicine has to contend with, is the escalating costs of drug and its development. For instance, to produce just one new drug can take years and cost millions. This accounts for the high and exorbitant costs of modern drugs. According to a report published by the US drug industry; an expenditure of some 58 million: US dollars is involved in the form of research and development costs, before a single new drug is introduced into the international market! All of this expenditure can take care of only about 20% of the population and that too, living mostly in big cities and towns. What happened then to the majority of the human population? Today, modern medicine with all its awe-inspiring progress; well-equipped hospitals, sophisticated research institutes, beautiful health care centres, multi-million and multi-national pharmaceutical industries, has gone out of the reach of the common man, who needs it most. While it caters only for the more affluent sections of the society even in the developed countries, the condition is simply deplorable in the developing and poorly developed countries of the world.

Definitely, modern medical practice has a lot of posers before it. It must therefore, as a matter of necessity rise up to the challenges of this decisive hour. For if it relinquishes its leadership in satisfying man's quest for health, humanity will naturally continue its forward march in search for a new alternative.

Criticisms against Modern Medical Practice

Critics of modern medicine have attracted public attention for their views that modern drug therapy, indeed modern medicine in general, does more harm than good. Others, while admitting some benefits from drugs, insist that this is medically marginal. In general, criticisms[4] directed against the medical profession are as follows:

Materialism/High Cost

Orthodox medical treatment is materialistic and tends to be expensive. In a depressed economy like Nigeria's, high cost of medical services seems to squeeze the remaining life out of poor patients. As the cost of modern health services increased, two kinds of medical services came into existence - one for the rich and the other for the poor. This contrasted sharply with traditional medicine, which is cheaper and sometimes the healers even prefer spiritual to material rewards.

Toxic Effect of Drugs and Side Effects

Certain drugs prescribed by the orthodox medical practitioner disrupt body's internal *milieu* (environment), producing lethal effects to other organs of the body. Sometimes these drugs produce adverse effects that are more harmful than the disease itself.

Invasive Methods of Treatment

Surgical operations," radiotherapy, organ transplantation, and so on, are considered very invasive, and sometime accidentally take their tolls on human lives.

False Claim of Completeness

In spite of the claim that modern medicine is holistic in its approach (that is, it has an answer to every problem), it's observed that in conditions where behavioural, emotional or spiritual factors play a major role, scientific method has comparatively produced less remarkable achievements.

Drug Abuse and Addiction

Dangers of drug addiction and abuse, which produce a sizeable number of psychiatric patients, are seen as negative effects and consequences of modern medicine to the human society.

Destructive Research and Emergence of New Diseases

Current biological warfare using potentially virulent micro-organisms (like anthrax) and the emergence of the AIDS virus are regarded as the consequences of modern science, which is the foundation of orthodox medicine.

Unholy Alliance with Pharmaceutical Industries

Orthodox medical practitioners are criticised for conspiring with pharmaceutical industries in either using human beings as experimental animals or exploiting them for mutual benefits.

Insensitive Bureaucracy in Patients' Management

Many patients criticise the long processes and procedures in the management of patients in orthodox practice. This involves long history-taking, clinical examination, series of investigations, co-management with other health workers, referrals, etc. In traditional medicine, there is 'no waste of time', as they say, in getting medical attention. It is easily accessible and available.

Prevalence Circulation of Fake and Expired Drugs

Many traditional healers consider the circulation of fake and expired drugs as the pitfalls of modern medicine.

Preoccupation with Disease and Neglect of Health

Modern medicine is often accused of its preocupation with the study of disease, and neglect of the study of health. Consequently, ignorance about health remains profound among orthodox practitioners. For example, the determinants of health are not yet clear; current definitions of health are elusive; and there is no single yardstick for measuring health. The credit to the decline in mortality is now more associated with health promoter factors (pure drinking water, clean environment and improved nutrition than to the awe-inspiring advances in modern medicine.

Medical Education in Orthodox Practice

Medical Education refers to the process by which individuals acquire and maintain the skills necessary for the effective practice of medicine.

Knowledge in Basic Sciences

To train as an orthodox practitioner or doctor, a person needs to have achieved a good level of understanding in the sciences (for example, physics, chemistry, biology), either at senior (high) school or at college. Medical schools are usually part of a university (although not all universities have medical schools) and they offer only a limited number of training places. This results in fierce competition for places, with only the best students being admitted.

Course Contents and Duration

In Nigeria, most medical schools offer a training course of about six years in duration. The curriculum is traditionally divided into two parts: a preclinical course in which the basic science of how the human body works is studied; and a clinical course in which the student is introduced to actual patient care in a hospital. The former is usually taught in science departments at the university and the latter at a hospital affiliated with the university.

The preclinical course involves such areas of study as the gross and microscopic appearance and connections of the human body (anatomy), the organisation and basic functions of different types of human cell (cell biology), the function and underlying biochemical processes of parts of human cells (biochemistry), the integrated functions of tissues, organs, and body fluids (physiology), the principal actions, distribution, and elimination of drugs in the body (pharmacology), the general principles underlying disease processes and such disease-related micro-organisms as viruses, bacteria, and parasites (pathology), the defence mechanisms of the body (immunology), and the structure and function of genetic material in living and infected cells (genetics).

The clinical part of the course involves medical students working with experienced doctors in general practice and hospitals to learn family practice and general medicine; and such specialised areas of health care as surgery (removal, reconnection, or transplantation of parls of the body), obstetrics (pregnancy and childbirth), paediatrics (diagnosis and treatment of childhood complaints), gynaecology (diagnosis and treatment of ailments of the reproductive system), geriatrics (diagnosis and treatment of ailments suffered by elderly people), and psychiatry (diagnosis and treatment of mental ill-health). During this time, medical students observe and learn from doctors working with patients on the wards and in specialist clinics, and gradually, under their supervision, become involved directly in the provision of health care (for example, diagnosis and administration of therapy).

Graduation and Administration of Physician Oath

Students have to pass examinations in all of these different aspects of the course, which take the form of written, practical, and oral tests. Upon graduating, they received a Bachelor of Medicine, Bachelor of Surgery (MBBS), or an equivalent degree. New doctors swear the Hippocratic Oath (or an equivalent professional statement) to adhere at all times to high standards of medical practice and ethics, and to protect the right of every patient to life, dignity, and confidentiality.

Internship and Supervision

It is usual for "junior" doctors to serve at least one year as an "intern" or "house officer" and to have responsibility for both diagnosing and treating patients in hospital. At this point, they choose to move away to a new hospital. Such a post, however, is considered to be an extension of their training with overall responsibility for their work resting with the senior colleagues supervising their work. However, the doctor receives provisional registration by the Medical and Dental Council of Nigeria (MDCN) which is supposedly to be renewed after a year.

National Service (NYSC)

After internship or housemanship, the doctor usually proceed for the compulsory one year national service through the National Youth Service Corps (NYSC) scheme, during which the doctor is exposed to the challenge of rural's peripheral practice and acquire more responsibilities. At this time, the doctor has received permanent registration from the MDCN as well as certificate of annual practising licence, which is renewable from time to time upon payment of a token.

Specialisation and Further Training

During his or her time as a junior doctor, an individual must decide whether to work in general or in a specialist branch of medicine. If the latter, the doctor applies to work with a particular specialist and his or her team, and once accepted, embarks upon a training course which lasts for several years; the training being obtained largely by the experience of working with other more experienced doctors in the group. During this time, he or she is called "registrar" or "intern" and the training culminates in both written, oral and practical exams set by an official body in that subject (for example, the West African College of Physicians/ Surgeons or the National Postgraduate Medical College of Nigeria) both of which decide whether a doctor is sufficiently knowledgeable and able to practise as a specialist in that particular area of medicine). If successful, the doctor is awarded "membership or fellowship" of the college, and designated consultant of the particular field.

Research and Career Development

It is important that doctors keep up with medical progress (the results of medical research concerning new forms of diagnosis and treatment). Most often, this takes the form of reading medical journals and books, attending conferences, and discussing medical matters with other specialists in the same or different fields. More recently, doctors have been able to communicate with one another and receive the latest medical information using the internet (often referred to as the "information superhighway"), which can link computers used by doctors in different hospitals and/or general practices around the world.

Hospital Clinical Meetings and Patients Care

Within the hospital set-up, it is customary for doctors to organise clinical meeting from time to time and make specific case studies of deaths and sickness of their patients. The aim is to review errors and consolidate on achievements. This is usually conducted openly with other members of the department or outside it who participated in the co-management of the patients. Ultimately, decisions are reached on improved patients' care and adopted for academic and administrative purposes.

Problems and Challenges

Over the last five decades, conventional medical education has thrived well in Nigeria with the number of medical schools increasing from one in 1948 to about 30 by 2003 and establishment of the National Postgraduate Medical College of Nigeria. Other achievements apart from the increasing number of Federal and state medical schools, including government financial support for education, improved teaching methodologies and participation of resident doctors, general practice orientation, confidence building and bilateral trusts, and cooperation of patients in the teaching process. In spite of these achievements, the following shortcomings are identifiable:

- That curative medicine has been emphasised more than preventive medicine and primary health care.

- Training of health personnel not geared to local conditions and resources.

- Inadequate community participation.

- Inadequate planning in respect of the socio-cultural and economic realities.

- Lack of adequate and up to date teaching technology and incomplete applied knowledge of the disease dynamics and the factors influencing health.

Other problems include absence of well-packaged continuing education-for-all physicians, lack of adequate indigenous philanthropy, accountability, cost effectiveness and productivity.

Presently, there is urgent demand for the refocusing of medical education in Nigeria in terms of detailed multidisciplinary planning within the context and realities of the country's socio-cultural and economic development. This again, as experts put it, is 'another call for Nigerian solutions to Nigeria's problems'.

Endnotes

1. In Nigeria, there are two (2) arms of this corporate body; namely a statutory arm represented by the Medical and Dental Council of Nigeria, the regulatory body set up by law; and the Nigerian Medical/Dental Associations, which are quasi-voluntary associations of all orthodox medical and dental practitioners in the land.

2. The three (3) primary learned professionals were the physician, the scribe (lawyer) and the priest.

3. This issue has been crucial in the history of orthodox practice. For example, reviewing some historical precedents, in 166 AD Galen fled Rome when plague struck the city. In 1665, Syndenham also fled London with the outbreak of bubonic plague. However, many physicians in Europe and North America have remained with their patients during various epidemics although their motivation was not always based on moral considerations. Sometimes, the outbreak presented an opportunity to improve status and income. A physician confronted with the need to care for victims of the plague confessed, "I to avoid infamy, did not dare remove myself but with continuous fear preserved myself as best as I could". In 1847, the American Medical Association (AMA) stated that; when pestilence prevails, it is the physician's duty to continue their labours for the alleviation of suffering, even at the jeopardy of their own lives.

4. These criticisms are not the personal opinion of the author rather the views expressed by many traditional medical practitioners, patients, the media and members of the general public (see Appendix VIII).

An Overview of Criticisms against Modern and Traditional Practice

Concerning the criticisms against modern medical practice, genuine as they may be, some of them are uncalled for. Medical science, like other branches of knowledge, has a lot of unsolved problems before it.

Pitfalls in clinical management sharpen the practitioner sensitivities and make him more humble in his quest for and parade of knowledge. *Drug abuse* tells of human inadequacies, *side effects* confess man's limitation in knowledge; *drug industry* speaks about the potentials to seeking for knowledge through research, trials and modification. *Long procedure and well thought decisions* in patients' care tell of meticulousness and diligence in dealing with human lives and *the demand for correct pay* speak of a legitimate demand for career advancement and material contentment to enable him attend to research and patients with 'one mind'. *Frequent seminars and publications* speak volume of the practitioners' readiness to share knowledge, learn from previous errors and improve on accomplishments in the course of practice.

As a result of all these, today modern medicine is not only international but multiracial having incorporated into itself the lore and legacy of many ages and societies. Yet, inspite of the gap, between modern and traditional medicine, which widens every hour, it is far better to build a bridge across the two arms. The traditional medical practitioner and his modern counterpart need to *come* to the negotiating table as colleagues and not as adversaries, provided they all agree to a common aim of alleviating human suffering and promoting the progress of humanity.

The current public view on modern health care delivery vis-a-vis elitist orientation, sophistication, limitations and so forth is a compound of vague expectation of 'miracle' cures with outrage when anything goes wrong. It is also a social demand for equitable distribution of health services. It is unreasonable to expect the public to be silence on these matters. Expectations has been raised and now, at the beginning of the 21st century with the manifest achievement of technology all around us, criticisms of the standards of modern medical practice may be justifiable. Even though expectation that modern medicine, as part of the technological package, must be perfect, is increasingly being portrayed as naïve. The public want benefits without risks and without having to alter its unhealthy ways of living; a deeply irrational position.

Again, there is a common misunderstanding of the fact that some impediments to health care delivery are politically and economically-induced as such outside the control of the medical profession. But it is easy to understand that a person, who has taken a drug into his body with intent to relieve suffering, whether or not it is self-induced, can feel profound anger when harm ensues.

Hence, the attitude of the modern medical practitioner that he has everything to teach others about health, disease and cure but nothing to learn from them, *is not just.* Such an attitude cannot be reconciled with wisdom, intellect, scholarship and the spirit of scientific inquiry. Similarly, the attitude of the traditional medical practitioner of viewing modern advances in medicine with contempt and disdain, his refusal to follow the trend of changes sweeping across the world and his preference to remain primitive amidst modernity is indeed condemnable. If the traditional healer, like the Okonkwo of Chinua Achebe's *Things Fall Apart,* refuses to move with the rest of the world, modern development will certainly bypass him *and our bridge may not avail him.* In this modern era, isolation, dissociation or insulation is considered illogical because virtually no individual, group or profession can exist independent of others.

No doubt, there is bound to be a gap of misunderstanding between traditional and orthodox practitioners, but this can be abridged by providing common forum for interactions and bilateral communication. It is true that modern medicine will continue to enjoy a superior status over traditional medicine because it is supported by advanced technology. However, it is also true that if the same technology is made available for research in traditional medicine, it will also attain its rightful place in alleviating the sufferings of humanity. Otherwise, the practitioner of traditional medicine in the modern world will continue to have difficulties in presenting his arguments for the advantages of his chosen therapy to the scientific and medical community.

Both traditional and orthodox practitioner have to agree that, it is the task of science (not doctors or pharmacists) to find the gems through conventional means from the wide varieties of healing practices and discard the dross, and at the same time, to leave intact socially valuable supportive aspects of traditional medicine. Even though, some may contend with the wisdom of validating or cancelling a medical or therapeutic system by means of another system. We need not to carry our contention too far, because scientific medicine is not dogmatic, it changes in accordance with evidence obtained by scientific enquiry applied with such intellectual vigour as is humanly possible. But this is not the case yet with some aspects of traditional practices. Thus, it is still rational to subscribe to a practice supported by evidence and experimental knowledge.

Perhaps, this is one of the strongest arguments against traditional medicine, that is, lack of scientific proof of the pharmacological properties of some of its medicaments. Surely for quite a long time, the traditional healers may not be in a position to provide scientific backing to their claims, but they should be encouraged. Clinical evidence of prolonged use of traditional drug without any observation of adverse effects should be provisionally accepted as evidence of efficiency and safety respectively. However, it must not be taken for granted that if a patient gets better when treated in accordance with certain practices, it is an evidence for the truths of such practices.

The blanket criticism of lack of precise dosage for traditional drugs is partly untrue. Nowadays, many healers do specify dosage using measures such as teaspoonful, cup, etc and even modify the dosage among different age groups. On the issue of unhygienic preparations of traditional drugs, this can be rectified through training and promoting awareness. The criticism against occult practices, witchcraft and magic cannot be explained away even by the most ingenious advocate of traditional medicine. Such methods cannot be verified scientifically and therefore are regarded quite rightly with suspicion and contempt by the orthodox practitioners.

Ideally even if methods differ, principles between the two systems must be shared and directed towards the good of the patient. But there are certain (evil) practices in traditional medicine that .tends to harm innocent persons. Such practices and beliefs must be condemned totally.

Other criticisms levied against traditional practice have to do with ethics regarding advertisement, arrogance, unwholesome rivalry and quackery. This issue should also be addressed. It is the duty of both the government and the practitioners themselves to salvage the profession from disrepute and abuse. If the various issues or criticisms raised are constructively addressed, the bulk of traditional healers could hold the prospects of providing additional source of health manpower particularly in rural communities.

On the other hand, many practitioners of traditional medicine charge that orthodox practitioners seems to neglect patients as whole integrated human beings (consisting of body, mind, and spirit) and treats them too much as machines consisting of several parts. Orthodox practitioners may well feel uneasily that there has been (and still) some truths in this, that some doctors have been seduced by the enormous success of medical science and technology and have become liable to look too narrowly at their patients and too easily to rely on a prescription where a much broader (holistic) approach is required. It is evident that such an approach is likely to give particular satisfaction in psychological and psychosomatic conditions for which orthodox doctors in a hurry have been all too ready to think that a prescription meets all the patients' need. In truth, a scientific approach in health care does not mean a patient must be treated as a mere biochemical machine or mean the exclusion of spiritual, psychological and social dimensions of human beings, rather it means treatments should be done in a rational manner.

The criticism that modern drug therapy does more harms than good, is a mere expression of disappointments or emotions rather than fair judgment. In spite of the many failures of modern therapy in treating chronic diseases and the consequences of side effects, carcinogens, drug-induced mutations, drug abuse and addiction, such accusations lack justification and fairness as such cannot be taken seriously. However, it is obvious that whenever a drug (whether traditional or modern, synthetic or natural) is taken, a risk is also taken. There are risks in taking medicines just as there are risks in food and transport. There are also risks in not taking medicines when they are needed, just as there are risks in not taking food or in not using transport when they are needed. In this case, people need to be advised not to disregard certain steps in seeking health care, namely; attending a health centre at the *right time,* meeting the *right people* (health workers, doctors, etc), getting a *correct diagnosis* of the situation, getting the *right prescription* for the required drugs, purchase of *genuine drugs* from certified drug stores and *appropriate use* of the drugs as duly prescribed.

Another important factor that is often ignored is the fact that people who use a particular drug are all likely to be different to some degree, either in their basic physiological make-up or in the circumstances surrounding the condition they are seeking to treat. Thus, an individual's response to a certain drug must be considered in isolation. When prescribed medicines are concerned, the practitioner interprets specific needs and situation and prescribes accordingly. There is now a growing trend to give an increasing share of the advisory role to the orthodox pharmacist who has years of training to qualify him to provide this all (very) important service. In the case of non-drug treatment or care of children, the aged and those who are too ill to cooperate, the role of nurses and social health workers is increasingly being employed.

The attack on the escalating cost of drug development is based on weak premises and claims which circulate only because they have not been challenged often enough. In spite of the huge expenses on drug development, it is fair to say that even if one percent (1 %) of active ingredient is found among many inactive plants through series of researches, it is indeed a great service to humanity in its quest for a better health.

Naturally, a discussion of this kind, which aimed at building a bridge of understanding between the two professions, must not overlook the fact that extremists exist in both sides. A difficult problem in communication is sometimes provided by the insistence of the traditional medical practitioner that the aims of his therapy must be qualitatively distinct from those of modern medicine. While the orthodox practitioner opposes the incorporation of traditional medicine into orthodox systems on the ground that providing medical care is too important, too complex and too dangerous to be left in the hands of untrained or differently trained personnel.

Generally speaking, there is no need for a conflict to occur.

The traditional healer would not have to turn his back on the experimental method rather than to the evidence of his own eyes, ears and patients. The scientific method does contribute to man's understanding of the world when used with enlightenment and true humility. It does not rest on acceptance of rigid and unalterable dogmas, and that it encourages opening new frontiers of knowledge for the good of all humanity.

Therefore, both the traditional healer and the orthodox practitioner have nothing to fear from integration. For the traditional healers, the legal recognition of their system of medicine as an official method of health care and the approaches outlined above will help to elevate them to a position of respect and social security.

For the orthodox doctors, emphasis must be made that an advocacy for integration or co-recognition of traditional medicine is neither an invitation to chaos in the health sector, nor is it to be mistaken or misconstrued as an excuse for shoddy or indiscipline practice, or an affront to medical profession. Rather, it must be noted that traditional medicine is being considered particularly in areas where modern medicine is not accessible to large populations for many reasons, and destruction of traditional medicine would leave unhappy, poor and sick people with nothing. One must also be mindful of the comments of the WHO on the role of traditional medicine where the facilities of modern health care are lacking. In other words, the WHO is supportive to programmes which evaluate and try to promote traditional remedies. That many of these remedies are of therapeutic value is no longer open to doubt, but the struggle is to ensure that they should be governed by the same standards of safety, efficacy and quality, as are required of modern drug therapy and practice. Here, one can make a plea that traditional and herbal remedies be considered in an even more positive light devoid of hostility and prejudices.

Any medicine, whether it is modern or traditional, is a science enriched by years of sacrifice. In the beginning, it may look more difficult or even impossible to consider the "good garbage" of traditional medicine for integration, but on continuation it will be found to be less expensive, less time consuming and more rewarding if properly planned. What it needs is careful thinking and re-organisation and the success of the endeavour will depend on able guidance and proper supervision, honest and intellectual approach and adequate financial aid.

Finally, it is hoped that an attempt has been made to revitalise the point that traditional medicine is worthy of consideration as a valid health care alternative in the modern world. It is to everyone's best interests to work together towards improving the quality of life and health everywhere in the world.

Prospects of Integration with Other Classes of Traditional Healers

It will be appreciated that there are varying classes of traditional medical practitioners in the country of which herbal medical practitioners constitute one single entity. It will be very difficult and unrealistic to propose that they should all be integrated into modern medical practice. For the meantime, as the traditional herbal practitioners seem to engage the attention of NAFDAC, pharmacists and pharmaceutical organisations, and other agencies, the following classes can be reassessed for possible integration.

- The Traditional Birth Attendant (TBA).
- The Barber-surgeon
- The Bonesetter
- The Religious healer

It is noteworthy that though the services of these categories of healers are extensively utilised by the people, many orthodox practitioners, without drawing a line of distinction between them, regard them as quacks and dangerous. They therefore, find it difficult to come to terms with them on the issue of health care delivery in the country. This may explain the existence of hostilities and grudges which each group harbour towards one another.

However, in spite of the derogatory and unwholesome attack on them by the orthodox practitioners, many people in the society still resort to them for treatment of their illnesses or when orthodox medicines fail to produce the desired results. In some rural areas, the traditional healers may be the only health care providers. Rural dwellers come into contact with orthodox practice once in a while when they visit the urban or semi-urban centres, when complication in a disease process has already supervened. The orthodox doctors, frustrated by the delays and by the harm done by such traditional healers, condemn them totally as 'harmful beings or at least useless additives in health care delivery'. The period before and in-between complications, in such emotional state is overlooked, which would have enabled the "little service" done by these healers to be appreciated, for example, the successful conduct of a thousand deliveries by the TBA, the circumcision of a hundred children by the barber-surgeon and the successful treatment of a couple of hundreds of people who presented to a traditional bonesetter with simple (uncomplicated) fractures or dislocations.

In view of the Alma-Ata Declaration which had recommended to governments the incorporation of certain traditional healers into orthodox practice in order to guarantee "Health for All" by certain period, more is expected from the orthodox doctor.

In fact, this group of traditional healers could serve as additional sources of health manpower in the country. This is a way the government could achieve a total health care coverage for its diverse communities and peoples. The traditional practitioners would, off course, need to be trained especially in simple hygiene, general modern concepts, health education, primary health care, locally endemic and epidemic diseases, first aid measures and simple emergencies, reproductive health, co-management with modern doctors or referrals and use of modern investigation techniques (like x-ray for bonesetters, packed cell volume for barber-surgeon, etc) and record keeping.

Viewed from another angle, the practice of primary health care involves a good deal of "de-professionalisation" of medicine, that is, allowing laymen to play a prominent role in the delivery of health care. While the physician still holds his unique position in the field of health care in general, the participation of other classes of workers (who are not 'professionals' in the present context) with relatively little training and support is an effective means of promoting health care delivery in the country. In this direction, it is not out of point to suggest that the traditional healer be considered as part of the "health team". It is indeed uncompromising that the ethics and standards of the profession be maintained and handed over to posterity *sine qua non*.

Therefore, as one orthodox medical practitioner rightly pointed out, "if sharing a table or title with another will make somebody to survive, the orthodox practitioners should have no qualms in doing so". But it is also a possibility that sharing such titles will also make another to die. However, an active participation of many orthodox practitioners in the evaluation and assessment of this and that category of traditional healer, is timely. Given the wide disparity in health care distribution, this will go a long way in eliminating the gap between the rich and the poor and between urban and rural communities with regards to health care delivery in this country. Such efforts, attention and participation will in due course be a rewarding project. It will increase the quality of health care provisions and/or coverage in Nigeria.

Furthermore, one may suggest that the prospect or possibility of integration of the above mentioned classes of traditional healers may lie in the fields of surgery, obstetrics, psychiatry and social medicine, so long as our quest for improved and wider coverage of health care service continues.

Herbal Medical Practitioners and the Role of NAFDAC

The use of herbal medicines can be said to be as old as man himself. They have been used in all societies for centuries. In spite of advances in modern medicine, and the introduction and widespread use of synthetic substances as pharmaceuticals, the use of herbs has survived till today. In fact, the demand and use of herbal medicines is receiving a great deal of attention in recent times in both developed and developing countries.

The WHO's declared target goal of "Health for All by the year 2000" in 1977 and the Alma-Ata Declaration on "Primary Health Care" in 1978 has drawn attention to the importance of herbal medicines particularly in the delivery of health care in rural communities. The policy adopted by the World Health Organisation (WHO) not only encouraged the development and use of proven traditional remedies in health care delivery system especially in the third world countries, but also placed the use of herbal drugs squarely in the areas of each government's public health policy.

The desire to use herbal medicine in modern therapeutics, calls for scientific identification, development and appropriate utilisation of herbs which provide safe and effective remedies in health care, so that herbal medicine can be absorbed into orthodox practice. However, before one talk of integration or co-recognition, the herbalist must be made to understand the importance of research, development and quality control of local drugs using modern techniques and applying suitable standards and good manufacturing practice. The herbalist occupies a central and indeed unique position among traditional healers, because he/she is a custodian of rich heritage in the use of herbal medicine.

In view of present policy of the government which recognises herbal traditional medicine and in particular encourages its development, a number of challenges lie ahead for the herbalists, the orthodox pharmacists, doctors, researchers and scientists. The Nigerian herbalists must rise to the challenges of improving their practice and maintaining discipline and professional ethics among themselves.

The NAFDAC must be ready to rise to the challenge of providing regulatory requirements and measures for the production and marketing of herbal medicine. This will go a long way in ensuring the safety, quality and efficacy of herbal drugs in circulation and available to the lay public for the treatment of minor ailments and to the health professionals for the treatment of major diseases as well.

The need to formulate appropriate public standards for Nigerian herbal products should take into cognisance the

WHO's guidelines or criteria which should be applied with due regard to local circumstances. The WHO has published "Guidelines for the Assessment of Herbal Medicines" which recommended the basic criteria for the evaluation of quality, safety and efficacy of herbal medicines. The guidelines provided information on

    i.   pharmaceutical assessment,

    ii.   product information for the consumer,

    iii. name of the product,

    iv. quantitative list of ingredient(s), v. dosage form,

    v.   indications,

        (a) dosage (if appropriate, specified for children and elderly)

        (b) mode of administration

        (c) duration of use

        (d) major adverse effects, if any

        (e) over-dosage information

        (f) contra indications, warnings, precautions and major drug interactions

        (g) use during pregnancy and lactation

        (h) expiry date

        (i) lot number

        (j) holder of the marketing authorisation, and

    vii. advertisement and other promotional activities to health personnel and the lay public.

It would be, as it seems to appear, a herculean task to regulate traditional herbal medical practice but assuredly, not impossible. The aim of regulation should be made clear to the herbalists, to ensure:

i. that the quality of the product is good and reliable at all times;

ii. that the medicine is safe, without any undue adverse effect now or on prolonged use;

iii. that the medicine is produced under acceptable circumstances that guarantee good manufacturing practice (GMP);

iv. that the product is packaged adequately and labeled with no misleading claims; and

v. that the medicines are distributed by qualified persons.

Surely, the traditional healers are not likely to be in a position to address all the regulatory requirements.

Nevertheless, they should be encouraged. Evidence of traditional use of a drug over a long period of time and without any report on dangerous side effects can be used to grant provisional acceptance of safety.

The fear of the herbal practitioner of not obtaining any tangible reward for making their knowledge public should be allayed by giving them some incentives. Any regulatory step to be taken must take into consideration the peculiarities of the various categories of producers and their products such that, traditional healers who casually prepare herbal remedies as the need arises for self-medication, home remedies or for their patients only (i.e. they are non-professional practitioners), should be allowed to continue to do so for now. Moreover, they can be helped to register their products provisionally so that information can be collected on the herbal remedies in the country.

Generally, efforts should be geared towards enticing the practitioners to present their products for registration, and they must be mobilised not to see the exercise as a punishment or sabotage against them. They should be made to appreciate the value of human life and the tragic consequence of losing health through the use of harmful drugs by a large number of people.

Being naturally gifted by a suitable tropical climate and fertile soil, Nigeria possesses a very rich flora and tropical plants. A great variety of plants grow in its forests, jungles, wastelands and in the roadsides. It is not surprising that many plants containing active and medical principles also grow abundantly within its bounds. Some 500 most important drug plants have been enumerated by Bep Oliver in his work on Nigerian medicinal plant. There are certainly many more of them growing in Nigeria. Almost all these indigenous medical plants are used extensively in the preparation of traditional medicines in Nigeria.

These plants also serve as important raw materials for many modern medicinal preparations. Since there has been no systematic survey of the medicinal plants of Nigeria, it is quite possible that many other potential medicinal plants in this country still remain to be explored and evaluated by research pharmaceutical institutions.

Finally, the government should provide the National Agency for Foods and Drugs Administration and Control (NAFDAC) the material and financial resources required for it to address the challenges arising from the development of herbal medicine in the country.

Regulation of the Medical Profession

The Medical and Dental Professions in Nigeria are regulated by the Medical and Dental Practitioners Act Cap 221, Laws of the Federal Republic of Nigeria (Decree No. 23 of 1988) which set up the Medical and Dental Council of Nigeria

(MDCN) for the regulation of medical and dental practice in Nigeria. The MDCN is a professional organisation that has the responsibility for licensing, training, and discipline of orthodox practitioners. It is the only institution with the authority to remove a doctor from the medical register.

Responsibilities of the Medical Council

The MDCN is charged with the following responsibilities:

1. Determining the standard of knowledge and skill to be attained by persons seeking to become members of the medical or dental profession and reviewing those standards from time to time as circumstances may permit;

2. Securing in accordance with provisions of the law, the establishment and maintenance of registers of persons entitled to practice as members of the medical or dental profession and the publication from time to time of lists of those persons;

3. Reviewing and preparing from time to time, a statement as to the code of conduct which the council considers desirable for the practice of the professions in Nigeria; and

4. Performing the other functions conferred on the Council by this Law.

By the provision of the law, the MDCN is empowered to make rules for professional conduct and established the Medical and Dental Practitioners Investigating Panel (MDPIP) and the Medical and Dental Practitioners Disciplinary Tribunal (MDPDT) for the enforcement of these rules of conduct.

Rules of Professional Conduct

The rules of professional conduct for medical and dental practitioners in Nigeria are made to enable medical and dental practitioners in Nigeria maintain universally acceptable professional standards or practice and conduct as well as to meet the demands of MDCN with regard to ethics and quality of professional practice.

These rules of conduct are meant to serve as guiding standards in the relationship of medical and dental practitioners with the profession, their colleagues, their patients, members of allied professions and the public.

Induction of a Newly Qualified Practitioner

By the rules, all newly-qualified medical doctors and dental surgeons shall be inducted formally into the profession at a ceremony during which the Registrar of the council administer the Physicians Oath to them and obtain from them the pledge to obey all the rules and regulations which guide medical and dental practices in Nigeria.

This ceremony is a solemn occasion during which the code of ethics of the profession is explained to new graduates and they on their part affirm publicly their commitment to abide by the norms, traditions and practices of the profession.

The Pledge by the Practitioner

The pledge which the new medical or dental graduate is required to make is in two consecutive parts namely:

(a) I, Doctor .... (the doctor being inducted publicly announces his/her name) do sincerely and solemnly declare that as a registered Medical/Dental Practitioner of Nigeria, I shall exercise the several parts of my profession to the best of my knowledge and ability, for the good, safety and welfare of all persons committing themselves to my care and attention, and that I will faithfully obey the rules and regulations of the Medical and Dental Council of Nigeria and all other laws made for the control of the Medical and Dental Professions in Nigeria.

(b) The Physicians Oath

Furthermore, the prospective practitioner also pledge to subscribe to the Physician Oath......... (see Appendix II)

The Disciplinary Organs of the Council

There are two disciplinary organs of the MDCN, namely:

1. *The Medical and Dental Practitioners Investigating Panel*

- The Medical and Dental Practitioners Investigating Panel is a court of first hearing in matters of alleged ethical misconduct that are properly brought before the MDCN.

- A doctor is required to be punctual whenever summon to appear before the panel in the course of the investigation of any case which involves him, whether as the defendant doctor or as witness.

- It is a grievous offence, subject to disciplinary action, for a practitioner, who has been duly notified that he has to appear before the panel in an ongoing investigation, to fail to appear whenever due, without an acceptable excuse. It does not matter whether he is within or outside the country.

•. The council may, if need be, communicate to a foreign medical council on disciplinary matters regarding any of her members who is deemed to be contemptuous of any of her disciplinary organs in order to assist them in treating the matter before them, in which he is involved.

2. *The Medical and Dental Practitioners Disciplinary Tribunal*

• The Medical and Dental Practitioners Disciplinary Tribunal has the status of a high court of the Federal Republic of Nigeria.

• Practitioner who appears before the tribunal whether as complainant, defendant or witness or represented by a lawyer is required to conduct himself as he would before a high court.

• The provision above is equally applicable to counsel who appear at the tribunal.

• Practitioner, who makes public comments on cases pending before any of the disciplinary organs of the MDCN or cases where the time for appeal has not expired, shall be guilty of contempt of the panel or the tribunal, as the case may be and shall be liable to appropriate disciplinary action.

5

The Way Forward

Today all over the world, there is renewed interest and attention to traditional medicine. This rousing trend is a reawaking on the role of traditional medical practitioners in modern health care especially in rural communities which constitute about 80% of the population in many developing countries.

In view of the socioeconomics and cultural status of developing countries, the magnitude of their health problems, rising population and extremely limited resources, many scholars have advocated for the integration and rehabilitation of traditional medicine in modern health care. The justification for this view is not far-fetched especially if one consider the following observations, that

- modern health care services is not equitably distributed throughout the world as only a minority of the world's six billion population have ready access to health services;

- most of the world's population depend on traditional medicine for health care services;

- the disparity and gross inequality in the health status of the people particularly between developed and developing countries, between the rural and urban communities as well as between the rich and the poor within the same country, widens every hour, in spite of the Alma-Ata Declaration of its "unacceptability";

- health care coverage is wider and more effective in areas where collaboration (in the form of integration or co-recognition) exist between orthodox and traditional practitioners than in areas where competition and confrontation is the norm;

- the bulk of traditional medical practitioners represent a potential workforce for health care delivery in rural areas;

- Africa, where large number of people die daily of preventable or curable diseases because of the lack of even simple health care, have the highest number of plant species in the world; and

- medical plants used by the traditional healers are of great importance to the health of individual and communities who are even eager to go back to nature for their health care.

Furthermore, the Alma-Ata Declaration on primary health care provided for the accommodation of proven traditional remedies in national health policies. Following the declaration and the activities of the WHO with regards to traditional medicine, many countries have sought for cooperation from WHO in identifying and using the safe and positive elements of traditional medicine in national health systems.

And because of its awareness that some elements of traditional medicines are beneficial while others are harmful, the WHO provided guidelines and criteria for the accommodation of proven traditional remedies in national drug policies and regulatory measures. It also encourages and supports countries in the identification and provision of safe and effective remedies for use in private and public health services. The WHO traditional medicine programmes has the following objectives:

- To foster a realistic approach to traditional medicines in order to promote and further contribute to health care;.

- To explore the merits of traditional medicine in the light of modern science in order to maximise useful and effective practices and discourage harmful ones; and

- To promote the integration of proven valuable knowledge and skills in traditional medicine.

Considering the socioeconomic situation in Nigeria and the frosty relationship between orthodox and traditional medicine practitioners (with some exceptions, of course) the integration of these two systems of medicine, in whatever form, will undoubtedly meet opposition from some quarters. However, efforts should be made by the government and the practitioners in the two professions to see that traditional medicine is examined critically and with open mind. The prevailing prejudice against traditional medicine should beset aside in order to attain the impartiality necessary to achieve the best in public health and to draw on all the resources of the nation - human and material, traditional and modern, for the greater benefits of the population.

In summary from the foregoing, it was recognised that in both developed and developing countries, the standard of health services expected by the public was not being provided. A very high proportion of the population in many developing countries, and especially in rural areas does not have ready access to health services. In short, there has been a growing dissatisfaction with the existing health services and a clear demand for better health care. Thus, despite the advances in modern medicine, traditional medicine is receiving a great deal of interest. This has been connected with many problems facing modern health care delivery in general. These are:

- Health facilities are few, far apart and inaccessible to the majority.

- The majority of the people are poor and cannot afford the services. The extreme poverty of the masses and all that this poverty is related to are highly detrimental to the health of the population.

- Even if the services are free, the cost of transport and time away from work are prohibitive. However, ignorance is a vital key factor here.

- Curative medicine has been emphasised more than preventive medicine and primary health care.

- Training of health personnel and technology is not geared to local conditions.

- The community participation is inadequate.

- There is inadequate planning which neglects multi-disciplinary approach within the context and realities of overall socioeconomic development.

It has been observed that many factors have contributed to making modern health care services inadequate to cater for the whole population. This situation, which depicts the glaring disparity on the state of health between developed and developing countries, urban and rural communities, and between the rich and the poor within the same society, have attracted worldwide criticism as a manifestation of social injustice. Concern for social justice and human rights has been the motivating force in fashioning a new approach to the basic human needs of the poor by calling for and working towards a more equitable distribution of health services.

With the present medical and scientific knowledge, and by exploring alternatives with relatively simple, low-cost appropriate measures, much improvement in health can be achieved.

Currently, the challenge facing the global community is to wipe out the inequalities in the distribution of health resources and services among peoples. In fulfilling this, the diverse health practitioners shall have to learn working as members of multidisciplinary teams and not be locked in their professional cells. This endeavour should, as a matter of necessity, involves and requires a good deal of 'deprofessionalisation' of medicine. Traditional healers and even laymen have a role to play in health care delivery. While the orthodox practitioner holds his unique position in the field of health care in general, the participation of a new cadre of health workers with relatively little training, orientation and support have to be considered. They shall now comprise part of the "health team". This arrangement shall be more applicable in rural areas of the developing countries like ours, where the practice and services of modern health care seems more of a utopia than practical reality. Thus, much rethinking and reordering of priorities will be necessary.

Therefore, in spite of the grave defects and deficiencies associated with traditional medical practice in Nigeria, it seems pertinent to conclude that the use, development and integration of some aspects of traditional medicine with modern medicine is important not only for the sake of advancement of knowledge and learning but also to meet the WHO urgent goal of health-for-all through the primary health care initiative which advocates a graded-level of health service that is always available, accessible, acceptable, affordable and effective in every community. This work is required even more in developing countries, because of the interplay of three factors:

i.   As an assertion of cultural identity,

ii.   As a means of escaping the increasing costs of modern health care services, and

iii. As a serious measurement of the efficacy of many traditional practices in the local setting, so that the rich herbage we possess can be adequately tapped for local purposes and export.

Therefore, it is essential to educate modern health professionals about the traditional medical practitioners, their methods, remedies, limitations and possible areas of development and cooperation. It must also be emphasised that traditional medicine, far from being outdated and primitive, conceptually provides modern medicine with many challenges and lessons to be learnt, although its practice continues to be rather crude and unrefined.

On the other hand, many a people as well as the traditional healers need to be informed about the giant strides and prospects of modern medicine. It is imperative for us to re-emphasise that scientific approach does not mean a patient must be treated as a mere biochemical machine nor mean the exclusion of spiritual, psychological and social dimensions of human beings. But it does mean treating these in a rational manner. As our knowledge of medicine continues to evolve and develop, gradually a more encompassing and comprehensive view of man, health and healing will be attained. This can be achieved by incorporation, through investigation and research, the best of all the different systems of medicine - traditional and modern - into one universal system for the benefit of mankind. This is the fervent hope for the future!

Recommendations

Finally, as a forerunner to a joint partnership, the following measures are recommended:

1. The government should establish a board or directorate of traditional medicine (in all the states of the federation) comprising orthodox medical practitioners, pharmacists and traditional healers, among others. The board shall be responsible for regulation, evaluation and registration of traditional medical practitioners.

2. The government should, through the said board, commission the compilation, standardisation and publication of approved formulation of traditional herbal drugs.

3. The board should ensure that some professional traditional practitioners establish a permanent station or traditional clinic where they can stay and operate.

4. The board should establish a college of traditional medicine and/or a herbal research institute in some of the universities in Nigeria.

5. The board should outlaw the aggressive, unethical, misleading, deceptive and self-sponsored advertise-ment by the traditional medical practitioners.

6. The orthodox medical practitioners should address the conflicts and issues or criticisms raised against them or the profession through agencies like the MDCN and NMAINDA.

7. The government should pay greater commitments towards ensuring an equitable allocation of health resources so as to make the atmosphere healthy, safe and protective for its citizens.

8. The non-governmental organisations and other charitable and voluntary organisations should assist in reducing or eliminating the existing gap among peoples in the distribution of health services.

9. The National Agency for Food and Drug Administration and Control (NAFDAC) should be empowered and provided with all the material and financial resources required for it to address the challenges arising from the development of herbal medicine in the country. The same goes for NIPRD and other pharmaceutical institutions whether in the universities or private establishments.

10. The board should liaise with the NAFDAC, Medical and Dental Council of Nigeria, the Pharmaceutical Council of Nigeria, and relevant organisations (national or international) in the discharge of its functions.

11. The board should encourage mutual understanding and exchange of information between the orthodox and traditional practitioners. Both practitioners should have basic knowledge of each other's profession.

12. The board should encourage members of the public and the media in creating awareness on the two systems while the infrastructure for monitoring, controlling and regulating them is being put in place.

References

Abdullahi, N. (2001) "Drug Preparation, Marketing and Use: A Pharmacological and Traditional Perspective." Seminar paper presented at the Opening Ceremony of the Annual Health Week of the Kebbi State Medical Students Association, Usmanu Dan Fodiyo University, Sokoto.

Akubue Iwe P. "Regulatory Requirements for Production and Marketing of Phytomedicines." A seminar paper presented by a lecturer of the Faculty of Pharmaceutical Sciences of the University of Nigeria, Nsukka.

Anonymous "Traditional Medical Practitioners and Specialists in Northern Nigeria - A Critical Analysis of Traditional Medicine and Evaluation of Possible Areas of Incorporation."

Babalola, A. (2001) "Medical Jurisprudence." Being text of a lecture presented at the National Executive Council meeting of the Nigeria Medical Association held at Ibadan, Nigeria.

Badoe, E.A., Archeampong, E.Q., and Jaja, M.O.A., (1994) (2nd ed): *Principles and Practice of Surgery in the Tropics Including Pathology.* Assemblies of God Literature Centre Ltd., Accra, Ghana.

Bannermen, R.H.O. (1979). "Acupuncture: The WHO View," *World Health* Magazine, December, pp. 14-29.

Bynum, W. (2004), *Medicine.* Retrieved on December 12, 2004 from Microsoft *Encarta Encyclopedia.*

Communiqué of the International Workshop on "Standardisation and Regulation of Herbal Medicines," organised by NAFDAC in collaboration with Bioresources Development and Conservation Programme

(BDCP) and the West African Pharmaceutical Federation (WAPF) held on 29th - 30th September, 1997 at Abuja, Nigeria.

Falase, A. O. (2001) (3rd ed), *An Introduction to Clinical Diagnosis in the Tropics.* Spectrum Books Limited, Ibadan, Nigeria.

George B. Y. (1983): "The Role of Traditional Healers in a Western-Scientific Medical System." *Nigeria* Magazine, No. 147.

Hanna, J. (2004) *Medical Law.* Retrieved on December 12, 2004 from Microsoft *Encarta Encyclopedia.*

Imobighe, T.A (1985) (edited) *Nigerian Defence & Security Issues and Options.* A Publication of the Department of Research, Nigerian Institute for Policy & Strategic Studies, Kuru, Nigeria.

Islamic Medicine Organisation and Kuwait Foundation for Advancement of Sciences. Bulletin of Islamic Medicine Vol. 2 Proceedings of the Second International Conference of Islamic Medicine, March-April, 1982.

Isezuo, (2001) "Man, Environment and Disease" in *The Journal of the Nigerian Medical Association,* Sokoto State Branch.

Iwu, M. M. "Production of Phytomedicines and Cosmetics from Indigenous Genetic Resources: From Lab to Market." Walter Reed Army Institute of Research, Washington, DC

John, T.A. (1997) (ed): *Medical Topics and Ethno-pharmacology for Traditional Medical Practitioners.* Proceeds of the 1st Workshop on Ethno-pharmacology and Traditional Medicine, organised by the WHO – Collaborating Centre for Traditional Medicine and College of Medicine of the University of Lagos in 1996 at Lagos, Nigeria.

Katzung, B.G. (1998) (7th ed) *Basic and Clinical Pharmacology.*

Large Medical Books /McGraw-Hill, US.

Lambo, J.O. (1979). "The Healing Powers of Herbs, with Special Reference to Obstetrics and Gynaecology," in *African Medicinal Plants* (ed. Sofowora, E.A). University of Ife Press, Ife, Nigeria, pp. 21-31.

Lawrence, D.R, Bennet, P.N & Brown, M.J. (1997) (8th ed') *Clinical Pharmacology.* Churchill Livingstone, US.

Lewis, C.E. (2004) *Medical Education.* Retrieved on December 12, 2004 from Microsoft *Encarta Encyclopedia.*

____(2004) *Complementary Medicine.* Retrieved on December 12, 2004 from Microsoft *Encarta Encyclopedia.*

MDCN (1995) (Rev. ed'): *Rules of Professional Conduct for Medical and Dental Practitioners in Nigeria.* Petruvanni Company Ltd., Lagos.

Meador, C.K. (1992). *A Little Book of Doctors' Rules.* Hanley and Belfus, Inc, Philadelphia, US.

Millan, C.A (2004) *Medieval Islamic Medicine.* Retrieved on December 12, 2004 from Microsoft *Encarta Encyclopedia.*

NAFDAC: Information Brochure on NAFDAC.

Naomesi, B. K. "Prospects for the Local Production of Phytomedicines." A seminar paper presented by a lecturer in the Faculty of Pharmacy, University of Science and Technology, Kumasi, Ghana.

Neal, M.J. (2nd ed.) *Medical Pharmacology at a Glance.* Oxford Blackwell Scientific Publication, London, UK.

Nkanginieme, KEO (1998) "Medical Education in Nigeria: The Perceived Blessings and Shortcomings." in *The Nigerian Journal of Medicine* Vol 7 No.2, April-June 1998.

NMA: The Constitution of the Nigeria Medical Association a$ adopted at the 2001 Annual Delegates' Meeting held at Benin City, Edo State, Nigeria.

NUMHP: The Constitution of the Nigerian Union of Medical and Herbal Practitioners.

Obiaga, P.C. *et al* (1999) (ed.) Conservation of Nigeria's Natural Resources and the Threatened Environment. Proceedings of the 26th Annual Conference of the Forestry Association of Nigeria held in Maiduguri, Borno State, 19th-23rd April, 1999.

Olaniyi A. A. & Adegbolagun O. M. (ed.) (1997): *Towards Better Quality Assessment of Drugs & Foods in the 21st Century.* Proceeds of 2nd National Workshop. Department of Pharmaceutical Chemistry, University of Ibadan.

Pamplona-Roger, G.D. *Encyclopedia of Medicinal Plants* Vol. I & II. Education Health Library. Editorial Safeliz, S.L.

Aravaca, Madrid, Spain.

Shehu, U. (1999). "Tuberculosis: The Challenges of a Resurgent Infection" in *The Nigerian Journal of Pharmacy,* Vol. 31, Jan-Feb, 2000.

Shehu, U (2002). Personal Communications: The Professor of Community Medicine, UNIMAID and Formerly, Sub-Regional Director, WHO.

Sofowora, A. (1993) (2nd ed.) *Medicinal Plants and Traditional Medicine in Africa.* Spectrum Books Limited, Ibadan, Nigeria.

WHO U978a) "Health Manpower Development: Training and Utilisation of Traditional Healers and their Collaboration with Health Care Delivery System." WHO Document No. EB 57/2.

WHO (1978b). "The Promotion and Development of Traditional Medicine." *Traditional Report Series,* No. 662, Geneva.

WHO (1989). "Traditional Medicine in the African Region."

Report of the first meeting of the WHO collaborating centres. Document No. AFR/TRM/4, Brazaville.

WHO (1991a). "Traditional Medicine and Modern Health Care: Progress Report by the Director General." Document No. A 44/10, 22 March, 1991. World Health Organisation.

WHO (l991b). "Guidelines for the Assessment of Herbal Remedies." Traditional Medicine Programme of the World Health Organisation, Geneva.

WHO (1992): "Review of the Traditional Medicine Programme (TRM)": WHO Document No. AFR/AR 42/19, Brazaville.

WHO (2004): Essential Drugs and Medicine Policy. Retrieved on December 5,2004 from http://www.who. int/medicines/.

WHO (2004): Report of the Consultation on AIDS and Traditional Medicine: Prospects for Involving Traditional Health Practitioners. Retrieved on December 5, 2004 from http://www.who.int/medicines/.

WHO (2004): Traditional Medicine: Growing Need and Potential. Retrieved on December 5, 2004 from http://www.who.intlmedicines/.

APPENDICES

Appendix I

Hippocratic Oath

I swear by Apollo the Physician, by Aesculapius[1], by Hygieia, by Panaceia and by all the gods and goddesses, making them my witnesses that I will carry out according to my ability and judgment, this oath and indenture (covenant).

To hold my teacher in this art equal to my own parents; to make him partner in my livelihood; when he is in need of money to share mine with him; to consider his family as my own brothers, and to teach them this art - if they want to learn it, without fee or indenture, to impart oral instruction, and all other instructions, to my own sons, the sons of my teacher, and to indentured pupils who have taken the physician's oath, and to no one else.

I will use treatment to help the sick according to my ability and judgement, but never with a view to do harm and injustice. Neither will I administer a poison to anybody when asked to do so, nor will I suggest such a course. Similarly I will not give to a woman an abortive remedy but will keep pure and holy both my life and my art.

I will not use the knife, not even, verily, on sufferers from stone, but I will give place to such as are craftsmen therein *(surgeons!)*. Into whatsoever houses I enter, I will enter to help the sick, and will abstain from all intentional wrongdoing and harm, especially from sexual relations with both female and male, be they free or slaves.

And whatsoever I see or hear in the course of my profession, as well as outside my profession in my intercourse with them, if it be what should not be published abroad, I will never divulge, holding such things to be holy secrets.

Now if I carry out this oath, and break it not, may I gain forever reputation among all men for my life and for my art; but if I transgress it and swear falsely myself, may the opposite of all this be my lot.

Physician's Oath[2]

(Modern Version of Hippocratic Oath)

I solemnly pledge myself to consecrate my life to the service of humanity:

I will give to my teachers the respect and gratitude which is their due:

I will practice my profession with conscience and dignity:

The health of my patient will be my first consideration:

I will respect the secrets which are confided in me, even after the patient has died:

I will maintain by all the means in my power; the honour and the noble traditions of the medical profession:

My colleagues will be my sisters and brothers:

I will not permit considerations of age, disease or disability, creed, ethnic origin, gender, nationality, party politics, race, sexual orientation, or social standing to intervene between my duty and my patient:

I will maintain the utmost respect for human life from its beginning even under threat, and I will not use my medical knowledge contrary to the laws of humanity:

I make these promises solemnly, freely and upon my honour.

Endnotes

1. Aesculapius (1200 Be) was an early leader in Greek medicine. Legend has it that he bare two daughters – Hygiea, who was worshipped as the goddess of health and Panacea, as the goddess of medicine. Aesculapius is still cherished in medical circles - his staff, entwined by a serpent continues to be the symbol of medicine to this day.

2. This is the Declaration of Geneva [Physician's Oath Declaration], adopted by the General Assembly of the World Medical Association in Geneva, Switzerland, in September 1948 and amended by the 22nd World Medical Assembly at Sidney, Australia in August 1968.

Appendix II

International Code of Medical Ethics

Duties of Doctors in General

1. A doctor must always maintain the highest standards of professional conduct.

2. A doctor must practice his profession uninfluenced by motives of profit.
    The following practices are deemed unethical:

    (a) Any self-advertisement, except as is expressly authorised by the national code of medical ethics.

    (b) Collaboration in any form of medical service in which the doctor does not have professional independence and/or free control over decisions on relevant professional issues.

    (c) Receiving any money in connection with services rendered to a patient other than a proper professional fee, even with the knowledge of the patient.

3. Any act or advice which could weaken physical or mental resistance of a human being may be used by a practitioner, only in the patient's interest.

4. A doctor is advised to use great caution in divulging discoveries of new techniques or treatment.

5.   A doctor should certify or testify to only that which he has personally verified.

Duties of Doctors to the Sick

1.   A Doctor must always bear in mind the obligation of preserving human life.

2.   A Doctor owes to his patient complete loyalty and the benefit of all the resources of his science. Whenever an examination or treatment is beyond his capacity he should summon another doctor who has the necessary ability.

3.   A doctor shall preserve absolute secrecy of all he knows about his patient even after the patient has died, because of the confidence entrusted on him.

4.   A doctor must give emergency care as a humanitarian duty unless he is assured that someone else is available to give such care.

Duties of Doctors to One Another

1.   A doctor-ought to behave to his colleagues as he would have them behave· to him.

2.   A doctor must not entice patients from his colleagues and must not conduct his affair in such a manner as to undermine their integrity.

3.   A doctor must observe the principles of The Declaration of Geneva '(the Physician's Oath).

Appendix III

Primary Health Care

With increasing recognition of the failure of existing health services to provide health care to all people and in all communities, alternative ideas and methods to provide health services have been considered and tried. In September 1978, at Alma-Ata in the former USSR, a joint WHO-UNICEF international conference attended by representatives of the governments of 134 countries and many voluntary organisations called for a revolutionary approach to health care, and a declaration was made, ever since, known as the Alma-Ata Declaration.

Declaring that "The existing gross inequality in the health status of people particularly between developed and developing countries as well as within countries is politically, socially and economically unacceptable", the conference called for acceptance of the WHO goal of health-for-all by the year, 2000 AD, and proclaimed primary health care (PHC) as way of achieving the goal. Though that utopian ambition has not been reached, PHC still remains the most effective tool of achieving the 'Health-For-All' target goal. The PHC lays emphasis on preventive and simple health care adopted to local needs and resources.

What is PHC?

PHC is defied as

> essential health care based on practical, scientifically sound and socially acceptable methods and technology made universally

accessible to individuals and families in the community through their full participation and at a cost that the community and country can afford to maintain at every stage of their development in the spirit of self-reliance and self-determination.

It forms an integral part both of the country's health system, of which it is the central function and main focus, and of the overall social and economic development of the community. It is the *first level of contact* of individuals with the national health system bringing health care as close as possible to where people live and work, and it constitutes the first element of a continuing health care process. PHC addresses the main health problems, including preventive, curative and rehabilitative services.

Essential Elements in PHC

PHC consists of at least eight elements, which are considered 'essential' and these are:

1. Promotion of effective nutrition;

2. Adequate supply of safe water;

3. Basic sanitation;

4. Maternal and child health, including family planning;

5. Immunisation against the major infectious diseases;

6. Education concerning prevailing health problems and methods of preventing and controlling them;

7. Provision of essential drugs; and

8. Appropriate treatment of common diseases and injuries.

Thus, PHC is a new approach to health care, which integrates at the community level all factors required for improving the health status of the population. It is based on principles of equity, wider coverage, individual and community involvement and inter-sectoral collaboration. Viewed in these terms, PRC is a radical departure from the conventional health care systems of the past. As a realisation of this, emphasis has therefore shifted from development of tertiary and curative care structures to the development of PHC interventions.

'De-professionalisation' of Medicine

The practice of PRC involves a good deal of "de-professionalisation" of medicine. It implies that health care delivery in spite of its unique importance must not be left in the hands of the professionals alone. Laymen have to come to playa prominent role in the health care delivery process. While the medical doctor still holds his unique position in the field of health care in general, the participation by a new cadre of health workers (for example, community health workers, traditional birth attendants, other practitioners of traditional medicine, social workers) with relatively little training and support have been considered and tried to provide or promote health care services. They now comprise part of the "health team".

Graded and Ladder-Step Approach

The aim of PRC is to provide all people in all communities of the world at least such a level of health that they are capable of working productively and of participating actively in the social life of the community in which they live. To achieve this, PRC takes into cognisance the "needs and ability" of individuals and communities. In this way, it provides graded and ladder-step services, some of which may not otherwise 'hold' in a more advantaged community. For example, in a remote rural area, *rice-water* or *carrot-soup* can be used in the treatment of diarrhoea and dehydration. Since the urge to 'do something' has always been the propelling force behind medical discovery, this can be grudgingly allowed. But as health services become readily available" as one move towards the urban settlements, the use of oral rehydration salts (ORS) or intravenous fluids cannot be compromised.

In this way, even though PHC attempts to eradicate the disparity in the distribution of health services and resources, it presupposes services that are both simple and efficient with regard to cost, techniques and organisation and which are readily accessible to those concerned, and that the individual, community and country can afford.

Appendix IV

Health Care Delivery in Rural Areas

Many people including health workers seldom appreciate the challenges faced by health professional working in rural communities. Medical problems, for example, in Suleja or Shagamu village differ greatly from those in Abuja or Lagos city. Though the basic approach to such problems may not differ in principle, they do in practice.

In general sense, there are practical differences between health care delivery in urbanised societies when compared to situations in rural communities. We need to face the reality of the situation by identifying these differences, which are largely due to hardships caused by poverty, deprivation, ignorance, cultural and socioeconomic circumstances.

In urban communities, there is relatively improved standard of hygiene and environment sanitation, fairly adequate supply of potable water, proper sewerage system, better housing and improved social amenities. The availability of all these facilities has conferred on those communities a remarkable uniformity in the overall pattern of disease and utilisation of health care services.

In contrast, most rural areas are poor, backward and deprived of many facilities that bear the hallmark of modem development. Consequently, rural dwellers still plagued by disease caused by poor sanitation, poor nutrition, poor water supply, poor housing, poor drainage and lack of awareness. Indeed, the majority of the patients who come to the rural health centres have diseases from such poverty.

As a result, it can be said that rural dwellers have not acquired the benefits achieved by their counterparts living in the urban and semi-urban areas.

Thus, the majority of patients in rural areas come from an environment where traditional healers enjoy a lot of popularity. Indeed, most patients seen in the hospital have already been through the hand of the traditional healers. They are the primary physicians in many rural areas and their medications may profoundly influence the course and presentation of an illness. Certain herbs concoctions and minor surgical procedures performed by these healers sometimes aggravate rather then alleviate the patient's illness. Yet, a rural dweller would rather consult a traditional medical practitioner in his own village than walk five miles to a health centre.

For those who pave not consulted the traditional medical practitioner, self-medication with homemade remedies or with drugs bought from open markets or chemist shops is the norm. Many patients therefore present in hospital when their diseases are already in an advanced, complicated or irreversible stage, or when the clinical picture is obscured by unguided interventions or therapies.

It can be rightly said that in most rural areas, the stages of seeking health care services by the local people is in a three-stage sequence; initial home remedy, then the traditional healer and lastly, orthodox medical practitioner, who bear the burden of the mishaps of others.

Another feature of health care delivery in rural areas is unconventional innovation. The use of simple low cost alternatives to conventional equipment, or using a piece of equipment for a purpose for which it was not designed are common, practices among rural health workers. This is because there are limited qualified staff, and dearth of equipment in most rural health centres or hospitals. The few equipment available may not function all the time because of lack of spare parts, maintenance expertise or adequate funding.

In addition, sophisticated laboratory investigations may not be available. Often, the patient may simply find that the drug prescribed may not be available in the locality or unaffordable. He may also find the procedure of going to the hospital as "too cumbersome" since he has to see several personnel' (cashier, medical records officer, doctor, nurse, pharmacist and laboratory technician) before medical attention is completed.

In rural areas, clinical default rate (that is, failure to comply with hospital appointment) is high. The patient may assume that an improvement in symptoms signifies a cure, which renders regular drug-taking and hospital re-attendance unnecessary. It is also not unusual to find that a patient who regularly keeps his appointment also regularly consults the traditional medical practitioner in his village. What more? He probably sees him more often than the orthodox health worker.

As in most developing countries, the patient-doctor ratio is low and the number of hospitals are inadequate. Consequently, the patient load is heavy and waiting time long. Yet, there are other problems that accompany a visit to the hospital such as the long distance, unreliable transport, rough road, and high fare. What else? On arrival to the hospital, the patient may find high cost of medical services which he cannot afford or could not have some laboratory investigations carried out because there is erratic or lack of power supply.

Health workerstrained in sophisticated teaching hospitals, whose organisation and facilities very often do not differ much from hospital in advanced countries. Those of them, who possess little or no experience in working in rural areas, may not realise that medical practice outside these institutions is markedly different. They may have to face the challenges of working in comparatively a frustrating or hostile environment. Rural health care providers must therefore decide upon a core set of inexpensive, available and alternative medicines to treat most of the conditions likely to arise in the course of their practice. Most often, they are on their own in deciding the sacrifices they have to undertake and the compromise they have to make in order to make health care services accessible and affordable to their host communities. This is one of the principles and cardinal objectives of the PHC.

Worldwide population growth and limited resources are today making health care in many countries analogous to the search for the 'golden fleece'. Many rural communities still face hardships caused by poverty, deprivation, cultural norms, and economic mismanagement, or disaster, both natural and artificial. In some areas of the world, where there is emphasis on commitment to local needs, traditional healers and orthodox medical practitioners have come to terms with one another and often work side by side, referring cases to each other. This is however, not so in other parts of the world like Nigeria.

Moreover, the' World Health Organisation in recognition of the important role traditional healers play in health care delivery in many developing countries is encouraging national government to incorporate certain practices along with the modern medical practices. Sooner or later, there is need for all health workers to address the challenge of rural health care delivery. While advocating for practical and realistic ways of addressing these challenges, it must be borne in mind that working in rural environment with myriad of problems can never be a substitute for discipline practice.

Appendix V

Health Care Delivery in the Military

By its nature, the military operates on land, sea and in the air. In other words, its area of operation encompasses all those areas that houses military personnel, whether temporarily or permanently (camps, barracks, etc), stationed or mobile, within or outside the country, and whether at war or during peace times. In other words, military environment is multi-dimensional since it can, and usually does, comprise areas that are not ordinarily habitable by civilian populations.

For the Navy, such an environment includes the ships whether at sea or at harbour just as the Airforce considers, although to a lesser degree, their flying or landed aircrafts or warplanes. Generally, in such an environment, it is indisputable that while health care maintains its basic concept of providing cure to the sick, the means and manner of approach will differ even if slightly with that in a "non-militarised" environment.

Naturally, the conventional means and facilities of providing health care may not always be readily available in a convenient form in such an environment. A comparative example is the case of providing first aid services to a wounded soldier in the battlefield (field first aid) and how that differs strikingly with the provision of such services to a common victim of road traffic accidents in the nation's highways. One must be quick to point out the difference which lies relatively in the absence of convenient and conventional facilities for such an endeavour.

Thus, even though during times of national disasters or major calamities, the challenge to any medical personnel could be as challenging as in any battlefield, military health care providers are usually confronted with situations quite different from those of their civilian counterparts. More often than not, they must, after satisfying the basic requirements, apply their own initiative and resourcefulness in handling situations arising from unusual or uncommon circumstances. In other words, they face a situation, which offers challenges that task the resourcefulness of the individuals concerned. The alternative could be the use of a core set of simple, result-oriented, effective, readily available and acceptable health care services to offer to their patients.

Hence, the means and manner of promoting effective health care services and its wider coverage in different categories of military operational environment remains a challenge to military health professionals. It has been noted for long that, research, study and utilisation of alternatives to conventional approach or using a piece of equipment for purposes other than which it was originally designed for as a life-saving strategy has become common feature of health care delivery in military environment. This is what the military will refer to as *"the way and manner strategy"* in problem-solving, provided the desired outcome is achieved.

Another aspects to this, is the inherent resourcefulness of the military vis-a-vis research and development. In fact, medical history has shown that many therapeutic (curative) breakthroughs are associated with discoveries made by early physicians while handling wounded soldiers in the battlefield. Therefore, the need to encourage efforts that will facilitate the harnessing of our national resources of men and material for an improved health care package for the military, whether at war or at peace times can not be over-emphasised. Fortunately, the World Health Organisation (WHO) has laid emphasis on the need for national policies that reflects local conditions and address peculiar health problems.

Thus, the need for the vigorous repositioning and reappraisal of this heritage through local research again cannot be over-emphasised. A re-appreciation of the intricate relationship and interplay between disease, environment and human initiative, calls for a concerted and co-coordinated planning in health care delivery between all the stakeholders involved. This is needed now, perhaps urgently, more than ever before.

The scenario of an uncoordinated operation of plural medical systems, in military sense is akin to a situation in which each arm of the country's armed forces fight it separate war. A level of coordination of various systems of medicine in the country is needed in order to avoid confusion in health care delivery, to minimise attendant negative consequences and to offer to patients the best in all the systems. An important obstacle to health care delivery is the problem of getting suitable skilled manpower and its subsequent development into desired specialisation. This is a common phenomenon confronting most armed forces in the world, since the military must compete with the industrial and public sectors for skilled manpower. The military being a more strict organisation is apt to be considered with certain apprehension due to inherent condition of the service, such as limitations of personal freedom, enforced· separation from home and family, and the physical risks and discomforts of many military duties.

Such considerations however tend to be biased and one-sided as they seems to ignore other conditions of military service which are encouraging and attractive namely, effective utilisation of individual skills and creative (research) abilities, opportunity for education, training and upward promotion, improved free medical care, housing and general welfare. In addition, considering the fact that the military generally is not a profit-oriented organisation but one that solely relies on government for its maintenance, there is an urgent need to encourage and support her health professional in exploring avenues in health care delivery that are simple, scientifically sound and inexpensive to maintain at every stage of the country's development in the spirit of self-reliance and self-determination.

At this period of Nigeria's developmental efforts and in view of the increased focus on professionalism, the military must intensify research aimed at harnessing our human, natural and material resources. As such exploring the various avenues in the field of traditional medicine and the integration of some beneficial practices holds a great potential for the future of health care delivery in the country. This however poses serious challenge to health care providers; as it will be a welcome addition to our armament in the war against diseases and suffering of our people.

It has often been stated that Nigeria is endowed with great human, natural and material resources. Emphasis should now be focus on harnessing these resources, and their effective utilisation for the betterment of humanity. The challenge is now before us to see that our country does not remain a consumer and importer-nation but a producer and exporter of our natural endowment as a contribution to mankind's quest for cure from diseases and 'medical disorders.

Guided by the conviction that the actual is more compelling than the potential and that one joule (ounce) of work is worth more than a tonne *of* speeches and resolutions, I painstakingly but hopefully committed myself to this work. Fortunately for me in this effort I received ample encouragement from the officers, men and civilian staff with whom I come into contact while carrying out my duties as medical officer at the Nigerian Navy Medical Centre, Borikiri at Port Harcourt. As a health professional, I do not see the military environment as a hindrance to creative zeal in research and promotion of learning. Rather, I see a lot of interesting challenges which could serve as a catalyst and a key to opportunities in acquisition of scientific knowledge and its application.

Finally, I must confess that this work, far from being the work of an expert is presented as a contribution by a health worker and an officer of the Nigerian Navy, who is conscious of his limitations in research, knowledge and experience in the field. I do hope that this humble effort will inspire experts (civilians and military) into further research in the subject for the purpose of improved health care package for all Nigerians.

Appendix VI

Traditional and Orthodox Practitioners: Relationship with the Media

In orthodox practice, the following rules guide relationship with the media.

(a) It is a long-standing tradition in the profession that doctor should refrain from self-advertisement. This has been so because of the appreciation by the profession that advertising could become a source of danger to the public in that, a doctor who was successful at achieving publicity might not in fact be the most appropriate doctor for a patient to consult. Advertising may also precipitate unwholesome rivalry among practitioners. In the extreme cases, advertising might raise hopes of a cure, which might prove illusory ..

(b) In view of the foregoing, a medical or dental practitioner would be deemed to have breached this code of ethics and would be found guilty of professional misconduct if he is proved:

   i.   to have advertised himself, whether directly or indirectly, for the purpose of obtaining patients or promoting his own professional advantage, or for any such purpose of procuring or sanctioning or aquiescenscing in the publication of notices commending or directing attention to the practitioners' professional skill, knowledge, services or qualifications, or deprecating those of others; or being associated with or employed by those who procure or sanction such advertisement or publication; and

ii.   to have canvassed, or employed any agent or canvasser, for the purpose of obtaining patients; or to have sanctioned, or been associated with or employed by those who sanction such employment, which are discreditable actions to the medical and dental professions and are contrary to the public interest.

Such a practitioner shall be liable to disciplinary actions.

Common Adverts Gimmick of Traditional Healers in Newspapers*

BE FREE FROM STAPHYLOCOCCUS

MEET

DOCTOR OF STAPHYLOCOCCUS

- Staphylococcus is a sexually-transmitted disease that destroys the reproductive organs and is responsible for causing breaking up of marriages as a result of sexual inadequacy by which a man cannot impregnate a woman. So to restore your sexual virility and fertility, consult .... *(name of the traditional healer)* the Doctor of all kinds of diseases.

- *Symptoms:* Itching in the private parts, general body weakness, severe waist pain, mucus on the penis, movement of worm round the body, acute pile, etc.

- *Effects:* Damage of reproductive organs, weak erection, watery sperm, low sperm count, and ultimately loss of sexual feelings.

- *Treatments:* You need *(name of the traditional healer)* no matter the number of years the suffering from 'STAPH', you will regain your sexual power again. Moreso, several practitioners have taken advice from me, they call themselves different names and claim to be experts in the treatment of STAPH. Though they may be good, but the master will always be the master. Don't delay, come to us as our prices are affordable. We assure you, you will be free from the diseases completely as you come.

  Our Address is .... *(address of the traditional healer).*

Appendix VII

Information on NAFDAC

The National Agency for Foods and Drugs Administration and Control (NAFDAC) was established by Decree No. 15 of 1993 as a parastatal of the Federal Ministry of Health. The functions of the agency include:

1. To ensure that food and drugs and other regulated products imported into the country meet the prescribed standards of safety, quality and efficacy;

2. To prevent the dumping of substandard and unwholesome products into Nigeria;

3. To ensure that local manufacturers of regulated products operate in accordance with the requirements of good manufacturing practice, and that their products meet acceptable international standards;

4. To combat the phenomenon of product faking and counterfeiting, a phenomenon that has assured international dimension and significance;

5. To ensure that regulated products particularly food products processed from primary agricultural materials are free from harmful chemical residues such as pesticide residues, etc.; and

6. To ensure that regulated products, particularly dairy products and sea food products are free

from harmful pollutants such as radioactive materials arising from nuclear accidents.

In the discharge of the above functions, NAFDAC assign specific responsibilities to three committees, six directorates, four units and some key organs.

Three main Committees

1. Finance and General Purpose Committee
2. Establishment and Disciplinary Committee
3. Technical, Research and Consultancy Committee.

Six Directorates

1. Administrative and Finance
2. Planning Research and Statistics
3. Narcotics and Controlled Substances
4. Regulatory and Registration
5. Inspectorate
6. Laboratory Services.

Four Units

1. Technical Services
2. Legal
3. Public Relations
4. Internal Audit.

Some Key Organs
For example, the Federal Task Force on Fake and Counterfeit Drugs.

Public Relations
NAFDAC maintains close contacts with the following organisations in Nigeria

1. National Drug Law Enforcement Agency (NDLEA)

2. National Institute of Pharmaceutical Research and Development (NIPRD)

3. The Pharmaceutical Council of Nigeria (PCN)

4. The Pharmaceutical Group of the Manufacturers Association of Nigeria

5. The Consumer Association of Nigeria

6. The Federal Environmental Protection Agency (FEPA)

7. The Standard Organisation of Nigeria (SON)

8. Other research Institutions in the Universities, etc.

International Organisations/Agencies

1. The United Nations International Drug Control Programme (UNIDCP)

2. The World Health Organisation (WHO)

3. The Codex Alimentarius Commission of the Foods and Drugs Administration

4. The Environmental and Occupational Health Science Institutions (EOHS).

Indeed, it is the duty of all governments to protect the health of their citizens. The challenge in this regard, apart from that of providing treatment facilities for the sick, is to prevent the hazards arising from .unwholesome foods, ineffective, substandard and adulterated drugs, toxic and corrosive cosmetics and chemicals as well as contaminated water.

Reflections and Observations

1. The activity of NAFDAC is an integral component of public health and preventive medicine.

2. Allover the world, particularly in developing countries, attention is being focused on preventive health because it is simpler and cheaper than curative measures.

3. All the agencies, directorates and committees of the NAFDAC seemingly direct their focuses on the organised system or segment of modern medical services.

4. Since the large-scale production of traditional medicaments seldom takes place, NAFDAC cannot officially recognise or register such products. .

5. Traditional healers and their drugs or herbs are now on rampage in the wider arm of the general society.

6. Logical deduction has revealed that more people patronise traditional medicine than modern medical practice in Nigeria. This implies that special attention is needed in the former without compromising the latter.

7. Most local handlers of foods and drugs in Nigeria, apart from institutionalised labour markets sector, are not effectively reached by the ambit of NAFDAC's control and regulation.

8. There is the need to empower the NAFDAC to decentralise its services to cover local and traditional herbs and packages (through the creation of a directorate of traditional medicine) and to establish more laboratories for evaluation of such local drugs and further research.

Appendix VIII

Questionnaire

(Assessment of Public Opinion on Traditional and Orthodox Medical Practice in the Country)

1. Name
2. Sex
3. Age
4. Marital Status
5. Literacy level
6. Locality
7. Profession/Occupation
8. Have you visited a traditional healer before?
9. If Yes/No, Why?
10. Have you visited a hospital before?
11. If Yes /No, Why?
12. What in your view are the problems associated with traditional medicine?
13. How do you think they can be remedied?
14. What in your view are the problems associated with modern medicine?
15. How do you think they can be remedied?
16. Do you have any remarkable experience with TM?
17. Do you have any remarkable experience with MM?

18. What is your observation about the relationship between orthodox and traditional practitioners in the country?

19. How do you view the advocacy for the co-recognition or integration of TM into modem health care services?

20. Which position do you advise government to take; co-recognition, integration or tolerance?

Index

149